Drug Resistant Infectious Diseases: Ethical Issues

Drug Resistant Infectious Diseases: Ethical Issues

Editor: Ezekiel Wilson

MURPHY & MOORE
www.murphy-moorepublishing.com

www.murphy-moorepublishing.com

MURPHY & MOORE

Cataloging-in-Publication Data

Drug resistant infectious diseases : ethical issues / edited by Ezekiel Wilson.
p. cm.
Includes bibliographical references and index.
ISBN 978-1-63987-170-4
1. Communicable diseases--Treatment--Moral and ethical aspects.
2. Infection--Treatment--Moral and ethical aspects.
3. Drug resistance--Moral and ethical aspects. I. Wilson, Ezekiel.
RC111 .D78 2022
616.9--dc23

Murphy & Moore Publishing,
1 Rockefeller Plaza,
New York City, NY 10020, USA

ISBN 978-1-63987-170-4 (Hardback)

Contents

Preface

The use of antimicrobials has increased to reduce illness and death from many infections, such as tuberculosis and pneumonia. The extensive use of certain antimicrobials and antibiotics has resulted in the development of drug resistance in the micro-organisms and has made these treatments less effective. Drug resistance occurs when the drug loses its ability to kill the micro-organism as a result of which the micro-organisms continue to grow and cause infection even in the presence of the drug. There are many pathogens that are drug resistant such as methicillin-resistant Staphylococcus aureus, carbapenem-resistant Enterobacteriaceace, etc. Staphylococcus aureus is resistant to several antibiotics. This book presents the complex subject of drug resistant infectious diseases in the most comprehensible and easy to understand language. It covers in detail some existent theories and ethical issues revolving around the drug resistant infections. Those with an interest in this field would find this book helpful.

Various studies have approached the subject by analyzing it with a single perspective, but the present book provides diverse methodologies and techniques to address this field. This book contains theories and applications needed for understanding the subject from different perspectives. The aim is to keep the readers informed about the progresses in the field; therefore, the contributions were carefully examined to compile novel researches by specialists from across the globe.

Indeed, the job of the editor is the most crucial and challenging in compiling all chapters into a single book. In the end, I would extend my sincere thanks to the chapter authors for their profound work. I am also thankful for the support provided by my family and colleagues during the compilation of this book.

Editor

1

Technological Fixes and Antimicrobial Resistance

Nicholas B. King

Abstract A 'technological fix' reduces the negative impact of a problem without addressing its underlying political, economic, or social causes. This chapter examines antimicrobials' central role in both the modern faith in technological fixes in medicine, and critiques of over-reliance on technological interventions that produce unintended consequences. The enduring appeal of technological fixes is rooted in their promise to provide simple, efficient, measurable, and effective solutions to complex problems; but this practically is purchased at the price of eliding important distributive concerns.

Keywords Ethics · Public health · Infectious diseases · Social policy · History of science

Introduction

In October, 2003, The Bill and Melinda Gates Foundation (BMGF) announced the first 14 'Grand Challenges in Global Health,' as part of an initiative to stimulate scientific research on diseases affecting less-developed nations. Grand Challenge #10 asked for applications that would help "discover drugs and delivery systems that minimize the likelihood of drug resistant microorganisms." In the intervening years, combatting antimicrobial resistance has continued to be a priority for the BMGF, with at least 50 grants funded through initiatives aimed at 'Creating Drugs and Delivery Systems to Limit Drug Resistance,' and identifying 'Novel Approaches to Characterizing and Tracking the Global Burden of Antimicrobial Resistance.' Funded projects include efforts to crowdsource surveillance of antimicrobial resistance (AMR), investigating the role of metabolic pathways in *M. tuberculosis*

N. B. King (✉)
McGill University, Montreal, QC, Canada

bacteria as a target for drug therapy, and identifying chemical entities that would act as 'selection inverters' to limit or reverse the development of AMR.

Given the problem's scale and complexity, the importance of developing technological solutions to improve surveillance and response to AMR might seem unassailable. However, soon after the initial announcement of the BMGF Grand Challenges, historian Anne-Emanuelle Birn published a sharp critique in *The Lancet.* Birn argued that, "in calling on the world's researchers to develop innovative solutions targeted to 'the most critical scientific challenges in global health', the Gates Foundation has turned to a narrowly conceived understanding of health as the product of technical interventions divorced from economic, social, and political contexts"(Birn 2005, p. 515). In the area of AMR, Birn argued that:

> Three more Grand Challenges addressing drug resistance and the development of cures for latent and chronic infections are also short-sighted. While access to effective immunotherapies for HIV/AIDS, tuberculosis, and other ailments has been appropriately termed a human right, integration of treatment with the well- established social and economic components of prevention surely merits at least one Grand Challenge. Here what deserves careful consideration are the factors associated with both HIV and multiple drug resistant tuberculosis: typically a combination of deprived social conditions—poor nutrition, overcrowded and unsanitary housing, economic insecurity, and inadequate health-care services—which lead to disease and can inhibit the taking of a complete course of medication (Birn 2005, p. 516).

Noting that "it is easy to be seduced by technical solutions"(Birn 2005, p. 516), Birn questioned the BMGF's assumption that the most pressing global health problems can be solved through the application of innovative scientific and technological solutions that target proximate causes of disease, while ignoring more distal political, economic, or social determinants of health. She concluded with a call for integrating both narrow technological and wider social interventions, and cautioned that "the longer we isolate public health's technical aspects from its political and social aspects, the longer technical interventions will squeeze out one side of the mortality balloon only to find it inflated elsewhere"(Birn 2005, p. 518).

Birn's general argument is commonplace in contemporary public health. These arguments frequently employ a critique of 'technological fixes' (or in Birn's language, 'technical solutions') – attempts to solve problems through technological innovations or interventions, without attending to the social, economic, or political factors that may have contributed to the development of the problem in the first place. Over-reliance on the promise of technological fixes has long been controversial in public health, particularly since the widespread recognition of the importance of the social determinants of health. Critics contend that too much emphasis is placed on 'downstream' technical solutions to health problems whose root 'upstream' causes are not amenable to technological intervention.

In this chapter, I will use the idea of a 'technological fix' as a window into the moral economy of responses to AMR, paying special attention to questions of distributive justice. Responding to antimicrobial resistance – which results from both a lack of appropriate medical technology and a complex web of behavioral, social, political, and economic factors – invites but also troubles the easy distinctions at the heart of the technological fix idea, and confronts us with difficult decisions regarding how best to distribute social and economic resources.

Technological Fixes

The idea of a technological fix arose within a context of postwar optimism that advances in science and technology could provide cheap and effective solutions to seemingly intractable social problems. While there were important precursors, one of the most important early popularizers of this view was Alvin Weinberg, a physicist and longtime director of the Oak Ridge National Laboratory. Weinberg had long advocated philosophical reflection and social awareness among scientists, particularly about the implications of 'Big Science.' During the 1960s, in a series of conversations with colleagues, he developed the idea that at least some pressing problems that were largely seen as intrinsically social might be amenable to simple technological interventions (Johnston 2018), culminating in an influential 1966 speech, "Can Technology Replace Social Engineering?" which was printed in a number of periodicals, including the *Bulletin of the Atomic Scientists*.

Weinberg argued that the causes of many pressing social problems of the day were intractably complex, and interventions targeting those causes are infeasible or impossible. He thus advocated remedies that can reduce or eliminate the harms generated by these problems, without addressing those causes:

> There is a more basic sense in which social problems are much more difficult than are technological problems. A social problem exists because many people behave, individually, in a socially unacceptable way. To solve a social problem one must induce social change – one must persuade many people to behave differently than they behaved in the past. One must persuade many people to have fewer babies, or to drive more carefully, or to refrain from disliking blacks. By contrast, resolution of a technological problem involves many fewer individual decisions (Weinberg 1991, p. 42).

Weinberg identified technologies that had already 'fixed' social problems, including the intra-uterine device (a 'one-shot' form of birth control which requires a minimum of individual motivation), development of safer cars (which reduces traffic deaths without having to improve driver competence), and even the hydrogen bomb (a strong disincentive to war that does not require greater tolerance or understanding). He proposed additional fixes, such as providing air conditioning to low-income households (to improve immediate personal comfort and potentially reduce rioting during hot summer months, without having to address the underlying social or economic causes of riots), and employing nuclear-powered desalination (which would eliminate water shortages without changing water consumer behavior).

While Weinberg was an admitted optimist and a tireless promoter of technological fixes, in his 1966 speech he struck a conciliatory note with potential critics: Noting that "technological solutions to social problems tend to be incomplete and metastable, to replace one social problem with another," he conceded that "we technologists shall not satisfy our social engineers, who tell us that our Technological

Fixes do not get to the heart of the problem; they are at best temporary expedients; they create new problems as they solve old ones" (Weinberg 1991, pp. 47–8). Answering the question posed in his title, Weinberg concluded that "technology will never *replace* social engineering...It is only by cooperation between technologist and social engineer that we can hope to achieve what is the aim of all technologists and social engineers – a better society, and thereby, a better life" (Weinberg 1991, p. 48).

Weinberg's hedging notwithstanding, his ideas about technological fixes met with immediate and sustained criticism; as early as 1970 the Oxford English Dictionary included wholly negative or ironic definitions of the term (Rosner 2004). Critics have mounted both practical and ideological objections. On the practical side, technological fixes provide at best short-term relief from the deleterious symptoms of social problems, but fail to address their root causes; at worst, they oversimplify intrinsically complex problems which they then fail to solve, and may introduce side effects that are worse than the problems they intend to solve. In a larger sense, the search for technological fixes is fundamentally reactionary in nature, encouraging society to seek cheap, quick, and partial solutions to holistic problems, while turning a blind eye to fundamental social and distributive injustices.

The transparent pursuit of technological fixes has had few defenders as vocal as Weinberg, and many detractors. This does not mean that the idea has fallen out of favor. Indeed, continued criticism is a sign of the enduring appeal of the idea of a technological fix, even if the term itself is not commonly used. For example, Evgeny Morozov's 2013 book, *To Save Everything, Click Here: The Folly of Technological Solutionism*, criticizes the 'there's an app for that' mentality of technological 'solutionism' in the internet age. Echoing earlier criticisms, Morozov argues that efforts to use internet-based technology to solve complex social problems – such as combatting obesity through exercise-tracking apps rather than food regulation – encourage us to define problems in terms of the technologies that might solve them, and discourage broader consideration of macro-level interventions (Winograd 2013).

Technological Fixes and Health

Technological fixes have been the subject of intense and sustained debate in the areas of public health and medicine. Advances in medical technology (e.g. vaccines, therapeutic drugs, surgical techniques, medical devices such as x-rays) play an undeniable role in diagnosing and curing disease, relieving suffering, increasing life expectancy, and improving population health. This fact alone would seem to justify continued investment of the BMGF Grand Challenges variety. Yet, beginning around the same time that Weinberg began evangelizing for technological fixes, critics began to question a similar logic underlying increasing investment in medical technology.

First, critics questioned whether medical advances played as great a role in health improvements as commonly believed. The classic statement of this critique is

Thomas McKeown's 1976 book, *The Role of Medicine: Dream, Mirage, or Nemesis?* McKeown argued that changes in political economy – including rising standards of living and better sanitation and nutrition – rather than specific therapeutic or preventive efforts, were responsible for the massive mortality declines of the ninteenth and early twentieth centuries (McKeown 1979). While the McKweown thesis has been hotly contested (Szreter 1988; Fairchild 1998; Colgrove 2002), it is now widely accepted that the contribution of technological innovation to historical improvements in health and longevity has been greatly overstated.

Critics also pointed to the unintended consequences of medical technology. The classic statement (and the 'Nemesis' of McKeown's title) is Ivan Illich's 1975 book, *Medical Nemesis: The Expropriation of Health.* Illich criticized medicine's role in the production of 'iatrogenic' illness, side effects of medical interventions that might often be worse than the original pathology they were intended to treat. He lamented the progressive "medicalization of life," which left individuals and societies ill-equipped to contend with normal aspects of human life including birth, pain, and death, as anything other than technologically-mediated pathology. And he objected to modern medicine's "radical monopoly" on all aspects of health and disease, diverting economic and intellectual resources from other attempts to improve the human condition.

Finally, critics contended that the pursuit of medical technology promoted a narrow approach to health and illness, rather than the environmentally and socially holistic approach that is actually necessary. In his 1959 book, *Mirage of Health: Utopias, Progress, and Biological Change*, René Dubos – a microbiologist who as early as 1942 had predicted the emergence of bacterial resistance (Moberg 1996) – argued that attempts to create a world free of disease are bound to fail, "because paradise is a static concept while human life is a dynamic process" (Dubos 1996, p. 281). Modern medical technology is ill-equipped to address the evolutionarily dynamic biological and social worlds, and single-minded pursuit of technological innovation is a fool's errand.

In the years since, the arguments mounted by McKeown, Illich, and Dubos have resonated with a wide variety of critics of technological fixes in clinical care, modern medicine, and public health. They have found most purchase among proponents of the social determinants of health, who contend that the majority of the world's inequalities in health result from political, economic, environmental, and social injustices, rather than lack of technological innovation. As the World Health Organization's 2008 report, *Closing the Gap in a Generation*, argues:

> Traditionally, society has looked to the health sector to deal with its concerns about health and disease. Certainly, maldistribution of health care – not delivering care to those who most need it – is one of the social determinants of health. But the high burden of illness responsible for appalling premature loss of life arises in large part because of the conditions in which people are born, grow, live, work, and age. In their turn, poor and unequal living conditions are the consequence of poor social policies and programmes, unfair economic arrangements, and bad politics. Action on the social determinants of health must involve the whole of government, civil society and local communities, business, global fora, and international agencies. Policies and programmes must embrace all the key sectors of society not just the health sector (WHO Commission on Social Determinants of Health 2008, p. 1).

Technological Fixes in the Context of Antimicrobial Resistance

It is no accident that Dubos developed his theories of microbial ecology, and his broader critique of the 'mirage' of modern medicine, within the context of his early work on bacterial resistance (Moberg 1996). Antimicrobials appear at first glance to be a technological fix par excellence, in the sense that they are a simple and effective technical solution to a complex problem with biological, social, political, and economic determinants. Indeed, a recent article critiquing the pursuit of technological fixes in dementia cited antibiotics as the classic case of a technological fix with unintended consequences (Jongsma 2017).

One could in fact argue that the apparent success of antibiotics is in large part responsible for a broader faith in technological fixes in medicine in the developed world. In 1967, during an oft-cited speech before American public health officials at the White House, U.S. Surgeon General William H. Stewart declared that it was time to close the book on infectious diseases and turn attention towards chronic health problems (Garrett 1994, p. 33). Stewart's optimistic claim reflects a perennial American faith in the power of biomedical science to conquer disease, but it is also evidence of a significant transformation in the burden of disease during the past century. In what is often referred to as the "epidemiologic transition," the proportion of deaths caused by infectious disease in the United States (and other industrialized nations) declined precipitously (Omran 1983). In 1900, infectious disease was responsible for 797 deaths per 100,000 population; by 1980, this figure had dropped to 36 deaths per 100,000 population. As mortality from infectious disease climbed, death rates for heart disease, various cancers, stroke, and accidents held steady or increased. In a dramatic reversal, chronic diseases replaced infectious ones as the leading killers in the United States. In 1900, 40% of deaths in the U.S. were caused by the eleven major infectious diseases (pneumonia, influenza, and tuberculosis alone accounting for more than 25% of all deaths), 16% by the three major chronic diseases (heart disease, cancer, and stroke), and 4% by accidents; by 1973, only 6% of deaths were caused by infectious diseases, 58% by chronic diseases, and 9% by accidents (Armstrong 1999).

The social and institutional ramifications of the epidemiologic transition were profound. Deluged with dramatic stories of patients snatched from the brink of death by antibiotics such as streptomycin and penicillin (dubbed "yellow magic" by Reader's Digest in 1943), Americans increasingly credited biomedical science for reducing the threat of infectious disease. This accelerated the transformation (or "narrowing"), underway since the early part of the century, of the focus of public health, from broad preventive measures towards clinical medicine, screening and the early detection of disease (Rosenkrantz 1974; Tomes 1998). This transformation was accompanied by changes in federal health expenditures as well: between 1950 and 1959, federal grants-in-aid declined from $45 million to $33 million, while funding for clinical and laboratory research jumped from $28 million in 1947 to $186 in 1957 (Fee 1994). The redirection of public and private funding from public health towards biomedical research would continue to accelerate into the 1980s, when it would be exacerbated by the dismantling of public health infrastructures in general under the pressure of Reagan-era budgetary constraints.

Even as much of the institutional apparatus for addressing infectious disease was being dismantled, the public and the medical profession increasingly mirrored Stewart's optimism regarding the threat of infectious disease. As historian Nancy Tomes notes, "With the array of drugs and vaccines available by 1965, the need to guard against contact infection understandably relaxed. Americans quickly came to believe that with a few soon-to-be-cured exceptions, modern medicine and public health had 'conquered' epidemic disease. Young physicians in the 1960s were advised, 'Don't bother going into infectious diseases,' and to concentrate on cancer or heart disease instead" (Tomes 1998, p. 254) Americans increasingly came to see infectious disease as a thing of the past, and they were bolstered in this confidence by the lack of significant epidemics of communicable disease – a confidence only briefly shaken by the HIV/AIDS epidemic, at least until the discovery of antiretroviral drugs.

Yet one can argue whether antibiotics truly 'fixed' the problem of infectious disease. As already noted, while they are often given full credit for the decline of infectious disease in Europe and North America, antibiotics were introduced after the majority of mortality declines that are more correctly attributed to rising standards of living, better nutrition, and basic public health preventive measures such as sanitation, vaccination, vector control, and provision of clean water (Szreter 1988; Cutler and Miller 2005). Moreover, social and economic factors continue to be major determinants of infectious disease (Semenza 2016). Even in high-income countries with well-functioning health care systems and access to a full range of antibiotics, poverty, social marginalization, and food and water quality continue to play a significant role in the incidence of infectious disease (King 2003; Semenza 2010). It remains to be seen whether, from a population perspective, investment in additional antimicrobials is the most effective or efficient way to reduce the burden of infectious disease.

Whether or not antibiotics 'fixed' infectious disease, their introduction generated the unintended consequence of antimicrobial resistance. While it might seem logical that a 'technological' problem (antimicrobials) demands a 'technological' solution (more antimicrobials), as the other chapters in this volume illustrate, the causes of and solutions to antimicrobial resistance are more complicated. As with infectious disease, the proximate cause of antimicrobial resistance is biological – pathogens develop resistance under the selective pressure exerted by use of antimicrobials – but underlying this proximate cause is a range of more distal determinants. These include, among others:

- Physician behavior – e.g., prescribing antibiotics for conditions caused by viruses (Sprenger 2015); engage in suboptimal practices such as use of monotherapy rather than combination therapy; and incorrect drug administration routes (Struelens 1998).
- Patient behavior – e.g., failure to complete full course of treatment; and self-medication, particularly in countries where antimicrobials are available over the counter.
- Poor hygiene, sanitation, and infection control in hospitals and other healthcare facilities, leading to cross-infection with multiple strains of bacteria (Aiello 2006; Struelens 1998).
- Widespread use – including misuse and overuse – of antimicrobials in agriculture (Levy 2014; Ventola 2015).
- Lack of development of new antimicrobials, which are less profitable than drugs for chronic conditions that are generally more expensive and used for much longer periods of time (Brown and Wright 2016).

Novel antibiotics will be introduced into the same social, political, and economic contexts that have contributed to the development of antibiotic resistance in the first place. Addressing these contexts would require, among other interventions: changing the behavior of physicians and patients to encourage appropriate stewardship of antimicrobials; instituting and enforcing new sanitation and infection control protocols at healthcare facilities across the globe; reforming an agricultural system dependent upon cheap antibiotics; and changing the incentive structure of the pharmaceutical industry to ensure that need rather than profit drives drug research.

Faced with a wide and seemingly insurmountable range of determinants, focusing on the development of new lines of antimicrobials through targeted research grants and incentive programs is attractive. Yet such a narrow pursuit would, ultimately, amount to little more than layering technological fixes on prior technological fixes. As Dubos noted a half-century ago, "Granted the obvious usefulness of sanitary practices, immunological procedures, and antimicrobial drugs, it does not necessarily follow that destruction of microbes constitutes the only possible approach to the problem of infectious disease, nor necessarily the best"(Dubos 1996, p. 53).

Technological Fixes and Distributive Justice

Technological fixes have an enduring appeal. Part of this is practical: they appear to provide simple, efficient, measurable, and effective solutions to complex problems. However, the presumed practicality of these fixes conceals underlying moral and political assumptions, with important ramifications for distributive justice.

One of Weinberg's precursors was Richard L. Meier, a chemist and technological optimist who advocated the use of technological systems as a means of eliminating poverty and other social ills (Johnston 2018). It is worth noting an important distinction between the little-known precursor and the widely-known successor: while Meier saw technology as a means of remedying distributive injustices, Weinberg saw it as a means for minimizing the harms of those injustices without addressing them. Indeed, in his influential 1966 essay, Weinberg's primary example of a successful technological fix is the advances in mass production of goods that "enable[d] our capitalistic society to achieve many of the aims of the Marxist social engineer without going through the social revolution Marx viewed as inevitable" (Weinberg 1991, p. 43).

The distinction between Meier and Weinberg illustrates an often-hidden ethical component of the technological fix approach. Technological fixes generally reward the rich. This is partially by design: fixes are appealing precisely because they avoid social engineering that might upset the status quo, including extant inequalities. They require no hard questions about the justness of current distributional procedures or outcomes, and they often expressly promise to reduce the negative consequences of extant inequalities without addressing the inequalities themselves.

The concentration of benefits among the rich is also a consequence of the global economy of health research. Health-related technological innovations are most likely to occur in wealthy institutions – top research universities, multinational pharmaceutical companies and medical device manufacturers, highly-capitalized biotechnology startup companies – concentrated in high-income countries. Initiatives that target technological innovation, from BMGF research grants to targeted incentives for pharmaceutical development, thus overwhelming benefit wealthy individuals and institutions in wealthy countries. While it is true that these investments may eventually benefit others, in the short-term they simply circulate resources from rich donors to rich institutions in the global north, often in the name of benefitting the least advantaged.

Technological fixes may thus be 'practical' insofar as they provide an easily identifiable, targeted, and efficient strategy for distributing resources; but this practically is purchased at the price of eliding important distributive concerns. In the context of antimicrobial resistance, we would do well to resist the urge to unthinkingly pursue technological fixes, lest they contribute to precisely the inequalities that underlie the spread of infectious disease and the continued generation of antimicrobial resistance.

Acknowledgments The author thanks Joy Tseng for research assistance in the preparation of this chapter.

References

Aiello, Allison E., Nicholas B. King, and Betsy Foxman. 2006. Antimicrobial resistance and the ethics of drug development. *American Journal of Public Health.* 96(11):1910–1914.

Armstrong, Gregory L., Laura A. Conn, and Robert W. Pinner. 1999. Trends in infectious disease mortality in the United States during the 20th century. *Journal of the American Medical Association* 281:61–66.

Anne-Emanuelle, Birn. 2005. Gates's grandest challenge: Transcending technology as public health ideology. *Lancet* 366:514–519.

Brown, E.D., and G.D. Wright. 2016. Antibacterial drug discovery in the resistance era. *Nature* 529(7586):336–343.

Colgrove, James. 2002. The McKeown thesis: A historical controversy and its enduring influence. *American Journal of Public Health.* 92(5):725–729.

Cutler, David. 2005. And miller, Grant. The role of public health improvements in health advances: The twentieth-century United States. *Demography* 42(1):1–22.

Dubos, Rene. 1996. *Mirage of health: Utopias, Progress, and biological change.* New Brunswick: Rutgers University Press.

Fairchild, Amy L., and Gerald M. Oppenheimer. 1998. Public health nihilism vs. pragmatism: History, politics, and the control of tuberculosis. *American Journal of Public Health.* 88:1105–1117.

Fee, Elizabeth. 1994. Public health and the state: The United States. In *The history of public health and the modern state*, ed. Dorothy Porter, 224–275. Amsterdam: Editions Rodopi B.V.

Garrett, Laurie. 1994. *The coming plague: Newly emerging diseases in a world out of balance.* New York: Farrar, Strauss and Giroux.

Johnston, Sean F. 2018. Alvin Weinberg and the promotion of the technological fix. *Technology and culture.* 59(2).

Jongsma, Karin R., and Sand, Martin. 2017. The usual suspects: Why techno-fixing dementia is flawed. *Medicine, health care, and philosophy.* 20(1):119–130.

King, Nicholas B. 2003. The influence of anxiety: September 11th, bioterrorism, and American public health. *Journal of the History of Medicine and Allied Sciences.* 58(4):433–448.

Levy, Stuart B., and Marshall, B. 2014. Antibacterial resistance worldwide: Causes, challenges and responses. *Nature Medicine.* 10(12 Suppl):S122–S129.

McKeown, Thomas. 1979. *The role of medicine : Dream, mirage, or nemesis?* Princeton, N.J.: Princeton University Press.

Moberg, Carol L. 1996. Rene Dubos: A harbinger of microbial resistance to antibiotics. *Microbial Drug Resistance* 2(3):287–297.

Omran, Abdel R. 1983. The epidemiologic transition theory. A preliminary update. *Journal of Tropical Pediatrics.* 29:305–316.

Rosenkrantz, Barbara. 1974. 'Cart before horse': Theory, practice, and professional image in American public health, 1870-1920. *Journal of the History of Medicine.* 55–73.

Rosner, Lisa. 2004. *The technological fix: How people use technology to create and solve problems.* London: Routledge.

Semenza, J.C., J.E. Suk, and S. Tsolova. 2010. Social determinants of infectious diseases: A public health priority. *Euro Surveillance* 15(27):1–3.

Semenza, J.C., E. Lindgren, L. Balkanyi, L. Espinosa, M.S. Almqvist, P. Penttinen, et al. 2016. Determinants and drivers of infectious disease threat events in Europe. *Emerging Infectious Diseases.* 22(4):581–589.

Sprenger, M. 2015. How to stop antibiotic resistance? Here's a WHO prescription.. Retrieved from http://www.who.int/mediacentre/commentaries/stop-antibioticresistance/en/

Struelens, M.J. 1998. The epidemiology of antimicrobial resistance in hospital acquired infections: Problems and possible solutions. *BMJ* 317(7159):652–654.

Szreter, Simon. 1988. The importance of social intervention in Britain's mortality decline, c. 1850-1914: A re-interpretation of the role of public health. *Social History of Medicine.* 1:1–37.

Tomes, Nancy. 1998. *The gospel of germs: Men, women, and the microbe in American life*. Cambridge, MA: Harvard University Press.

Ventola, C.L. 2015. The antibiotic resistance crisis: Part 1: Causes and threats. *Pharmacy & Therapeutics*. 40(4): 277–283.

Weinberg, Alvin M. 1991. Can Technology Replace Social Engineering. In *Controlling Technology: Contemporary Issues*, ed. W.B. Thompson. Buffalo, NY: Prometheus Books.

Winograd, Terry. (July 1, 2013). What's wrong with technological fixes?: Boston review.

WHO Commission on Social Determinants of Health. 2008. *Closing the gap in a generation: health equity through action on the social determinants of health*. Final report of the Commission on the Social Determinants of Health. Geneva, Switzerland: World Health Organization, Commission on Social Determinants of Health.

2

Antimicrobial Resistance and Social Inequalities in Health: Considerations of Justice

Lynette Reid

Abstract Within-country social inequalities in health have widened while global health inequalities have (with some exceptions) narrowed since the Second World War. On commonly accepted prioritarian and sufficientist views of justice and health, these two trends together would be acceptable: the wealthiest of the wealthy are pulling ahead, but the worst off are catching up and more are achieving sufficiency. Such commitments to priority or sufficiency are compatible with a common "development" narrative about economic and social changes that accompany changes ("transitions") in population health. I set out a very simple version of health egalitarianism (without commitment to any particular current theory of justice) and focus on two common objections to egalitarianism. Priority and sufficiency both address the levelling down and formalism objections, but these objections are distinct: giving content to equality (I argue here) places in question the claimed normative superiority of priority and sufficiency. Using examples of the role of antimicrobials in both these trends – and the future role of AMR – I clarify (first) the multiple forms and dimensions of justice at play in health, and (second) the different mechanisms at work in generating the two current patterns (seen in life course narratives and narratives of political economy). The "accelerated transition" that narrowed global health inequalities is fed by anti-microbials (among other technology transfers). It did not accelerate but replaced the causal processes by which current HICs achieved the transition (growing and shared economic prosperity and widening political franchise). The impact of AMR on widening social inequalities in health in HICs will be complex: inequality has been fed in part by tertiary care enabled by antimicrobials; AMR might erode the solidarity underlying universal health systems as the well-off seek to maintain current expectations of curative and rehabilitative surgery and chemotherapy while AMR mounts. In light of both speculations about the impact of AMR on social and global health inequalities, I close with practical and with theoretical reflection. I briefly indicate the practical impor-

---

L. Reid (✉)
Department of Bioethics, Dalhousie University, Halifax, Canada
e-mail: Lynette.Reid@dal.ca

tance of understanding AMR from the perspective of health justice for policy response. Then, from a broader perspective, I argue that the content by which I meet the formalism objection demonstrates that the two trends (broadening within-country inequality and narrowing global inequality) are selective and biased samples of a centuries-long pattern of widening social inequalities in health. We are not in the midst of a process of "catching up". In light of the long-term pattern described here, is the pursuit of sufficiency or priority morally superior to the pursuit of equality as a response to concrete suffering – or do they rationalize a process more objectively described as the best-off continuing to take the largest share of one of the most important benefits of economic development?

Keywords Bioethics · Public health ethics · Antimicrobial resistance · Health inequality · Health justice

Introduction

What is the significance of antimicrobial resistance (AMR) for health inequalities? This question refers not just to the extent to which AMR might exacerbate or mitigate health inequalities, but to the ways that we should think about health inequalities in order to be adequately sensitive to the justice dimensions of AMR and to the lessons that AMR might offer about the nature of health inequalities as such and their normative status (or the normative plausibility of responses to health inequalities).

The development of AMR in bacteria, viruses, fungi, and parasites detrimental to human health is already a substantial public health concern; it is estimated to cause 700,000 deaths a year globally. The UK government's O'Neill report paints what it calls a worst-case scenario—a post-antimicrobial world in which antimicrobial-resistant infections are collectively the second leading cause of death by 2050, causing 10 million deaths a year and lowering world population by 700 million (O'Neill 2014, 2016). This "worst case scenario" is based on projecting the consequences of AMR for a small selection of conditions and as such may underestimate the potential consequences of AMR (Jamrozik and Selgelid, Chap. 1, this volume).

It is widely acknowledged that the development of AMR will have different effects on high-income, middle-income, and low-income countries. Other chapters in this volume propose or evaluate policies to address and mitigate AMR as these matter for health equity and for global health.

In this chapter, I situate the use of antimicrobials and the growth of AMR in a narrative of population health (Valles 2018), specifically the story of narrowing global (between country) and widening local (within country) health inequalities, and argue that the development of AMR puts pressure on normative commitments to sufficientism and prioritarianism as purportedly more feasible and more normatively satisfying goals for health justice.

Faced with data showing that people who live in one neighbourhood may have a life expectancy 10–20 years lower than people in a nearby neighbourhood, or that the difference in life expectancy between countries is in some cases as high as 35 years, many express a normative worry that social inequality in health and global health inequalities are unjust (Marmot 2015). However, among academics who discuss health justice, few are egalitarians about health. Sufficiency – the attainment of a decent minimum – is often argued to be an appropriate goal; priority for the worst-off is argued to be adequately action-guiding. The question of sufficiency, priority, or equality can be deferred to ideal theory; we need not agree on an ultimate goal in order to act. For example, if we can agree that AMR is likely to hit the worst-off the hardest, as the O'Neill report projects, then sufficientists, prioritarians, and egalitarians alike can focus their attention on alleviating its effects for the worst-off while still remaining faithful to their diverging commitments if they wish.

Health Inequalities and Health Egalitarianism: Definitions

In this chapter, I use the term "social inequality in health" to refer to inequalities in some health indicator across socioeconomic status (SES) or other category of interest to justice within countries. I will refer to life expectancy or mortality, but metrics of inequality include other key indicators, for example, infant mortality or workplace mortality. I will use "global health inequality" to refer to inequality in such indicators across low-, middle-, and high-income countries (typically referring to LMICs on the one hand and HICs on the other).[1] Granted that there is normatively significant variation in what counts as socioeconomic status and how it is measured, I speak broadly of socioeconomic inequalities in health, while not intending any specific version of the concept as fundamental. (I motivate/explain this below.)

The core commitment of a health egalitarian is that, all things being equal, a society in which persons of different socioeconomic status can lead full lives with minimization and mitigation of health-related disruptions to those lives is more just than a society in which the possibility of a healthy life is patterned by

[1] The less cumbersome phrase "health equality" refers simply to the distribution of life years across a population, not correlated with any other variable of interest to justice. For example, Strømme and Norheim recently claim that both global and national health inequalities are shrinking (Strømme and Norheim 2017). They base this claim on a univariate measure of the distribution of a health indicator alone (age at death) within a population: their empirical claim is that the distribution of age at death is becoming more closely clustered around a value rather than spread widely or polarized while their implicit normative claim is that form of health inequality is what matters to justice. Such univariate measures of health inequality, however, capture nothing about who is dying early or late within that narrower distribution – for example, the rich or the poor, the racialized or the non-racialized, those of higher or lower educational attainment, or all social classes equally (Regidor 2004). Life expectancy could cluster around a given value without any change in the gap between the rich and the poor.

socioeconomic status. That is, a society in which service workers, manual labourers, or those excluded from labour market participation live lives as long and healthy as executives or professors is more just than a world in which this is not the case. On a global scale, a world in which such possibilities of health are not patterned by accident of global birth is more just than a world in which that is not the case.

Following Temkin (2000, 2003), I explore the health egalitarian commitment without assuming a specific view on whether this commitment should dominate feasibility considerations or other values that may conflict with the achievement of social equality in health or global health equality. For example, a commitment to cultural self-determination may outweigh a commitment to health egalitarianism in specific cases, granting the moral and political right of a community to pursue economic activity and social organization that exposes it to different supports for and risks to health, such that life expectancy differs from that obtained in urban settings in HICs.

The leveling down objection seems particularly acute for health egalitarians: while it may be acceptable to take financial resources from people for redistribution, can it ever be acceptable to worsen the health of some people in order to achieve some increment of improvement in the health of the less well off? Temkin's approach avoids the common use of this "leveling down" objection (Parfit 1997, 2012) to take egalitarianism off the table. We can explore the normative importance of social equality in health without *ipso facto* committing ourselves to the view that it has such normative weight that it trumps other considerations and values.

Toward a Multi-dimensional Account of Justice, Health, and Equality as a Normative Goal

A health egalitarian faces (at least) three substantial challenges: the leveling down objection (discussed in the previous section), the challenge that health inequalities *qua* natural can only be matters of justice insofar as they cause or are caused by unjust social inequalities, and the challenge of motivating normatively a concern with the abstract and interpersonal measure of inequality. These three challenges – the leveling down objection, the natural difference objection, and the formalism objection – are closely related. For example, one might focus on concrete normative concerns – suffering (and its alleviation) or sufficient health (and its achievement) – and, by adopting prioritarianism or sufficientism, avoid both the formalism and the leveling down objections (as in Anderson (1999, 2010) and other proponents of capabilities (Nussbaum 2006; Venkatapuram and Marmot 2013)). However, these objections are conceptually distinct. Filling out the concrete realities that are reflected in formal measures of inequalities might bolster rather than undermine the case for equality over sufficiency or priority as a normative goal.

In this paper I use examples drawn from antimicrobials and antimicrobial resistance to give content to concerns about social equality in health, showing that the formalist challenge can be met without adopting a sufficientist or prioritarian alternative to egalitarianism. I do not offer or adopt a specific comprehensive theory of justice or even of justice and health; rather, using examples from antimicrobials and antimicrobial resistance, I explore different forms of justice and different relationships between justice and health. These are phenomena that an adequate account of health justice should capture, but what account of health justice in what form will do that adequately is not a question I attempt to resolve here.[2]

Certainly, injustices in domains other than health affect health outcomes; health states lead to injustices in other domains (e.g. fair opportunity, strict equality, reward for merit, reciprocity, respect for privacy or property, etc.). For these reasons, judgements of justice and injustice in other domains inform the normative evaluation of the justice or injustice of social inequalities in health and global health inequalities. But health needs also constitute specific claims for recognition, in response to which we should, as a matter of justice, express respect for equal human worth. That is, health inequalities, in addition to causing and being caused by other unjust inequalities, also constitute and express specific relations of equality and inequality that are of concern to justice.[3]

Furthermore, unequal responsiveness to health needs creates social inequalities that are *sui generis* and that are politically significant in *sui generis* ways. Consider that the inability to access medical treatment that could address a serious health condition creates desperation which may motivate people to enter into social relations they would not otherwise contemplate. For example, in moral reasoning tests, psychological researchers ask participants to evaluate a scenario in which a person needs a medication they cannot afford for their fatally ill spouse. This is the paradigmatic case in which otherwise socially unacceptable actions become reasonable and moral responses to inequality.

My pluralism about forms of justice is not in the first instance motivated by the idea that liberal public policy must avoid commitment where individual moral views diverge. Any claim to neutrality is dubious. Rather, it is an acknowledgement that conceptions of justice and fairness can take different contextually-relevant forms (e.g. fair reward for effort; fair opportunity; recognition of achievement; acknowledgement of and response to need), as can oppression (e.g. economic exploitation; exclusion from wealth or resource base; denial of voice). Inequality or oppression in any of these forms may be produced by other inequalities that themselves raise question of justice, and may produce further such inequalities. As Wolff and

[2] This complexity may not be captured by a "spheres of justice" view, where a given domain of human endeavour is governed by a single form of justice (Walzer 2008). Consider that educational policy must be responsive both to the importance of reward for merit and to the importance of equal opportunity for achievement of a reasonable standard of literacy for citizenship and fulfillment. No education system only rewards achievement or only brings the population to whatever minimal or reasonable standard can be achieved by all.

[3] Sen (2002) makes something like this point about the concept of health *equity* as a multi-dimensional concept: there are several forms that equity takes in relation to health and in relation to matters that have bearing on health and all of these must be taken into account in a treatment of health equity.

da-Shalit have argued, injustices that compound in these ways may be of particular concern (Wolff and da Shalit 2007).

Answering the formalist challenge involves contextualization and narrative exploration to evaluate the significance of what is portrayed in health statistics. The relevant narratives include individual lives (life-course narratives) within the context of social structures and broad changes in those structures – i.e. narratives of political economy. Both population level narratives of political economy and individual narratives of life courses contribute to understanding the human and normative significance of broad epidemiological changes in longevity and the social and global equality and inequality in these measures.

Examples

In this section, I show these multiple relations of health and justice by taking two examples from microbial disease, antimicrobials, and AMR.

Example: AMR, Sex, and Gender

Women's health as measured at the population level is strongly influenced by sexual and reproductive health, and these are in turn conditioned by reproductive autonomy or its absence, as a matter of technology and crucially as a matter of gender politics. (The influence of perinatal experiences on population health measures is substantial; to be discussed below.) At the level of individual life narratives, childbearing is a normative, but of course not a universal, experience for women.

Antibiotics are used prophylactically in childbirth to address the risk of maternal and infant morbidity and mortality from infections. I have been unable to locate in the medical literature discussion of the implications of AMR for obstetric practice, such as discussion of whether prophylactic use constitutes a sustainable form of anti-microbial stewardship, under what conditions it might be abandoned by choice or triaged by need, or what the implications of its waning efficacy would be for women's health. Neither have I been able to locate discussions of the implications of AMR for handling the infections that will be more common if the efficacy of prophylactic antibiotics is lost. Presumably this would have a significant impact on women's reproductive health.

Childbirth is normative for women but not universal – many women give birth and there are cultural expectations whose negotiation characterizes women's lives whether they themselves give birth or not. There are different pathways by which women come through sexual intercourse to childbirth, with greater or lesser degrees of autonomy and under different conditions of gender-related and economic justice and injustice. Sexual assault is both a concern of justice as a criminal matter and a concern of political justice, insofar as it is an expression and a tool of gender-based domination. The sequelae of sexual assault sometimes include health and social effects (e.g. sexual transmitted infections, pregnancy, trauma, altered social standing, and deep effects on current or future intimate relations, exposure to a criminal justice system that may be partly or entirely inadequate to victims' needs, etc.); these have further health and social effects (infection in childbirth, to return to the original example).

Some of the health-related harms of sexual intercourse are harms that we have been able to mitigate with antimicrobials (e.g. gonorrhoea, HIV/AIDS, infections arising from termination, infections arising in childbirth) for the last decades. These will be affected by AMR. Noting substantial disagreement about the moral and political status of sex work, sex workers and/or persons subject to sexual exploitation will be particularly affected by AMR. Some will take this as compounding the injustice of sexual exploitation and others will take it as compounding the injustice of the stigmatization of sex work. As such, AMR will alter the experience of sexual activity and affect concerns of justice in relation to sexual activity.

Example: AMR and Parasitic Infection

Hookworm is a parasitic infection caused by inadequate public health infrastructure (Pilkington 2017). It is virtually unknown in HICs; the United States is an exception to this, which may not be surprising given that it boasts the highest GINI co-efficient (greatest economic inequality) of HICs and captures a low proportion of its national income (30%) for state expenditure (Piketty 2014, pp. 475–6). Anthelmintic resistance (resistance to the anti-parasitic agents used in treatment) is a growing concern for hookworm (Harhay et al. 2010).

The conditions for hookworm arise directly from the legacy of indentured labour on large estates where land was held by a small elite, and so it is strongly conditioned by historical injustices in colonial and slave-holding societies. As a hygienic disease it is tied closely to place, and place is tied closely to identity for many groups subject to colonialism – whether they were brought as slaves to work in a place that is now home or they experienced colonial occupation and seizure of their lands, transforming their status as labourers on those lands.

In turn, hookworm has health sequelae detrimental to participation in the labour market and fulfillment of care responsibilities in the home (McKenna et al. 2017) and so it also has forward-looking intergenerational effects that are of concern for justice and the perpetuation of relations of economic inequality in post-colonial societies. This compounds the historical colonial relations that gave rise to the risk exposure.

These injustices are compounded by the fact that there is little or no investment in research to tackle this problem. Instead, anthelmintic drug development serves the agricultural industry, with the goal of increasing efficiencies in food production for the better-off, rather than serving the medical needs of the worse-off – human beings who live in conditions that make them vulnerable to the parasite (Hu et al. 2013).

Summary of Examples

In these examples, justice concerns and health inequalities are intimately and complexly linked. A given health advantage or detriment can reflect justice or injustice in gender relations, in criminal justice matters, in labour relations, in global economic and colonial relations involving claims to land, resources, and sovereignty – in addition to the common justice-related concerns about the fair distribution of scarce resources within health care.

The forms of stigmatization to which infectious and hygienic disease are subject are paradigmatic and concrete forms of stigmatization. Shame involves the source of the infection (in sexual relations, or in place for historically constituted communities consigned to exposure to hygienic disease) and this extends to shame about the resulting health state, in ways closely tied to disease-related identities, to symbolic and quasi-symbolic stigma (denigration, shunning, isolation, social distancing) and to concrete stigmatization (violation of civil liberties, detention; situating waste disposal on "unproductive" land where this is land occupied by indigenous and poor communities).

AMR has its effects in these fields. As it renders infectious and hygienic diseases less susceptible to treatment, it will exacerbate the ongoing legacies of these historical harms and their forward-reaching effects, in part by compounding the relevant health effects, and in part by the effects of policy responses on marginalized populations. For example, persons exposed to STIs through sex work or sexual exploitation and persons exposed to hookworm through colonialism and its legacy of land marginalization may in turn be subject to increased state surveillance and control, even risk of criminalization, insofar as their health state is seen to pose a threat to others, or insofar as their health state gives them a claim resources that increasingly come to be seen and managed as scarce public or common goods (Smith and Coast, Chap. 17, this volume; Giubilini and Savulescu, Chap. 9, this volume).

In describing the examples, I draw on (not very detailed) meso-level narratives in which justice considerations abound – narratives that involve local manifestations of broader structural relations for specific communities. In these narratives, it is relatively clear how justice considerations relate to health and how health differentials can intrinsically constitute the justice or injustice of relevant relationships. But what connection can we draw from here to the broadest population metrics of health inequalities? What roles have antimicrobials played in these population narratives and what role might AMR play?

Health Inequalities: The Development Narrative

Recall the 10–20 year within-country differences in life expectancy between high- and low-income neighbourhoods and the 30–40 year differences in life expectancy between HICs and LMICs. Do the differences among groups captured in the population health metrics matter normatively, and are they a concern of justice? What role did antimicrobials play in generating these differences and how might AMR affect these differences?

Now, these formal measures might matter because those at the low end of the distribution are experiencing health deficits which we want to address as a matter of beneficence, or as a reciprocal obligation to supply a decent minimum arising from our economic inter-dependence – or they might matter because the *inequalities* of which they form one extreme matter. It is easy to elicit some kind of normative concern about these inequalities but much more difficult to specify exactly what matters about them as inequalities. Two persons might have different life expectancies because of accident or genetic endowment; it's not obvious why group differences matter. One possible starting place is the thought that if all else were equal the poor would be as healthy as the rich. That is, the poor do not constitute a separate natural kind with different potential to be healthy. If they are differentially unhealthy, it is because we fail to ensure that everyone has access to their potential to be healthy, because incomes are inadequate, housing poor, food of low quality, work hazardous, childbirth ill-supported, and access to care and social support for recovery from ill health limited. This line of thought is similar to the view of that health inequalities matter to justice when they are caused by or cause other injustices, but it maintains at its core the idea that health inequalities matter as such and can constitute injustice.

By analyzing the role of antimicrobials in broad trends for social inequality in health and global health inequality, I argue that understanding the causes and the narrative constitution of these trends renders sufficientism and prioritarianism less attractive as normative stands.

A common account of the broad trends in both global health and economic development in recent decades is that within-country inequalities are widening, but between-country inequalities are narrowing – a narrowing that is particularly dramatic since the 1950s for health and 1980s for economic status. The normative claim attached to this account (implicitly or explicitly) is a prioritarian or sufficientist claim that while things may look grim from the perspective of the middle classes of HICs, from the perspective of those who are truly the worst off, things have never looked better: more and more people in the world are relieved of the worst form of poverty ("absolute poverty") and are achieving a sufficiency of health. In health, the worst off are doing even better: life expectancy is advancing faster than it did when the current HICs built their prosperous economies over the course of the nineteenth and twentieth centuries.

In the examples of the previous section (16.3), I outlined different ways that justice questions might reflect, be reflected by, or otherwise enter into health inequalities, by tying life course narratives to narratives that matter to justice – political and cultural economy, including gender relations. In the same manner, I will approach the significance of population health metrics in relation to justice by exploring the meaning of these metrics in terms of the typical and divergent life courses of the members of a population and in terms of the political and cultural economy of the communities in question (within-country communities and global communities).

The common narrative reflecting the sufficientist or prioritarian reading of narrowing health inequalities is the development narrative (political economy) linked to life course narratives via "transition" theory (demography and epidemiology).

Demographers long ago observed the tendency of populations to pass successively through certain stages, tied to their economic development: populations move from having a high birth rate along with a high death rate (in foraging or pastoral economies), to a more stable and dropping death rate, while the birth rate remains high, resulting in a population explosion (from agricultural to early industrial economies), to a low birth rate-low death rate stage, which we see in the stable or shrinking populations of modern HICs (which depend at this stage on immigration for economic growth). Epidemiologists in the mid-twentieth century linked these demographic changes to patterns of health and disease: the first stage of "pestilence and famine" with its characteristic population swings is followed by a second stage of greater stability but low life expectancy conditioned by infectious and hygienic diseases, initially from the close co-habitation of animals and humans and then the increasingly crowded, eventually urban, living conditions of humans with one another. With improvements in living standards and public health infrastructure, we enter a third stage where chronic ("man-made and degenerative") diseases of later middle age emerge as common causes of death (Omran 1971). A combination of so-called lifestyle changes (e.g. smoking cessation, moderation of red meat consumption) and advanced medical technologies (e.g. cancer treatment) have pushed back these diseases of midlife and created the ongoing extension in lifespan that HICs are now experiencing, which some describe as a "fourth stage" of epidemiological transition (Olshansky and Ault 1986).

These are the economic and epidemiological narratives behind how a non-transparent metric like life expectancy is read in health policy and understood to be a normative concern or a concern of justice. A life expectancy in the 40s reflects substantial maternal, infant, and child mortality caused by infectious and hygienic disease and the lack of empowerment of women to control their sexual and reproductive lives. A life expectancy in the 60s reflects a society in which heart disease and cancer are leading causes of death in later middle life, a phenomenon that emerged over the course of the twentieth century in HICs. A life expectancy in the 80s reflects improved prevention and treatment of these major killers and the emergence of new common forms of dying in advanced old age, e.g. frailty and dementia.

The dramatic narrowing of global health inequalities since the 1950s is called, within this narrative, the "accelerated transition," reflecting the success of the international development agenda in achieving improvements in health status that outstrip the economic and political development of the countries in question – that is, that outstrip both growth in GDP and changes in the franchise and effective political organization of workers to demand the health, education, and safety benefits of modern welfare states. By these means, industrialization and urbanization raised GDP while political change led to a larger proportion of the GDP being invested in the well-being of the population, in a process that involved the empowerment of workers and women, improving population health – although (given the dynamics of democratic pressure) achieving less success in addressing the needs of so-called minorities.[4]

On this narrative, it seems natural to see the changes in global economic and health equalities and inequalities in terms of the idea that some countries got a head start and some lag behind. A common economic belief is that open markets and the transfer of skills and technology will ensure that LMICs continue to advance towards (eventually) "catching up." The common narrative in health is that some (both low and high tech) public health technologies could be transferred in advance of economic development, offering LMICs a leg up in the development process.

Is the Development Narrative True?

Is this development narrative true? Does it do the normative work it claims to do?

One important critique of formal measures of equality and inequality is that they are not transparently related to the underlying realities they measure (King et al. 2012; Harper et al. 2010; Mackenbach 2015, Mackenbach et al. 2016). King et al. point out that the same underlying reality can be represented as a narrowing of absolute inequalities or a widening of relative inequalities, for example. Similarly, the same numeric change may represent different causal pathways or encapsulate different social relations with different significance in terms of justice and injustice and different distributions of well being and suffering. This has implications for the normative concern that these measurements might inspire (which inequalities should we tackle?) and may even raise questions about the reality of abstract interpersonal measures (are inequalities simply imposed on the individual phenomena that, sufficientists and prioritarians argue, should be the object of our moral concern?).

Underlying Realities

The narrative that LMICs are "catching up" suggests that they are achieving what HICs have achieved, but doing so later. However, this suggestion is false. The accelerated narrowing of global health inequalities represents fundamentally different epidemiological patterns, causal pathways, and relations of concern to justice.

[4]In the current HICs this process led to the state capturing 40–55% of national income for its spending (Piketty 2014, pp. 475–6).

I described above how a population's life expectancy in a given decade is "read" epidemiologically, and I noted that many different underlying patterns of health and disease can generate the same measure. Substantial infant and early childhood mortality in a subpopulation might depress life expectancy as much as widespread exposure of young adults to interpersonal violence, workplace hazards, tuberculosis, or HIV. Different narratives of political economy can in turn generate these patterns – the sub-population with elevated early childhood mortality may be indigenous or migrant; interpersonal violence may be a matter of warfare or the combination of lack of opportunity, crime, availability of guns, policing, and racialization.

The picture offered by transition theory is simplified (Frenk et al. 1991; Defo 2014). Researchers now emphasize that the same life expectancy in different populations may reflect different realities. They describe the transitions of LMICs as "incomplete" transitions, highlighting counter-transitions within LMICs and even within HICs. For example, LMICs did not leave infectious and hygienic disease behind. Rather, they are taking on the so-called diseases of affluence – diseases that arise from changes in work, nutrition, energy, and transportation – in addition to carrying an on-going burden of infectious and hygienic disease (Santosa et al. 2014; Defo 2014). Specific population groups within HICs experience the re-emergence of infectious and hygienic disease, while the emergence of so-called "diseases of despair" (suicide and substance abuse) may reverse health gains in HICs for some groups (Case and Deaton 2015) or for entire countries (some of the former eastern bloc). Global migration resulting from instability and lack of opportunity in LMICs and the need for low-wage workers particularly in the agricultural sector in HICs brings together the AMR diseases of LMIC and the population health profile of HICs (Suk et al. 2009).

Furthermore, insofar as LMICs have substantially reduced childhood and young adult mortality from infectious and hygienic diseases, these reductions did not come from the developments in political economy that led to such improvements in HICs. In HICs, rising GDP went along with political changes (universal suffrage extending beyond male property owners to labourers and women, and various political movements organized around these identities) and these brought about improvements in determinants of infectious and hygienic disease. In HICs, antibiotics joined and accelerated an existing process of decline in infectious and hygienic disease after the Second World War (Mackenbach 1996). In LMICs, on the other hand, growth in GDP resulting from urbanization has not been distributed or re-distributed and invested to improve living standards and public health infrastructure to the same extent. Political empowerment is limited, in part by the actions of the very same global corporations that bring (some) growth in income to LMICs. In its place, a global network of health philanthropy has delivered effective prevention with vaccines and mosquito nets and treatment with antimicrobials for infectious and hygienic diseases that remain endemic. Antimicrobials played an important role in this so-called "accelerated" transition. The infectious and hygienic diseases that result from crowding and exposure to waste are managed medically e.g. by vaccination for prevention or by antimicrobials for treatment, and not by improved housing for primordial prevention. This is not a lag in economic development or in the uptake of health-related technologies; it is a different path of economic and social change. Even to describe it as "incomplete" is misleading, insofar as the term "incomplete" suggests that LMICs have reached a different point on the same pathway instead of achieving the partial benefits they have achieved from a different trajectory.

This is evident at the level of life course narratives. What a life expectancy of 60 looks like in a current MIC is not what a life expectancy of 60 looked like when HICs reached that stage. Parents in HICs may feel that childhood and adolescence are times of risk and danger, but very few children in HICs experience life-threatening diarrhea or pneumonia and virtually no adolescents and young adults experience TB. (The exceptions to this general picture are in communities within HICs that bear a heavy burden of colonialism such as indigenous communities (Orr 2013 and Møller 2010) and in the globally mobile working class (MacPherson et al. 2009), where migration is also conditioned by colonial histories in addition to current global supply chains.) Parents in LICs with superficially similar mortality figures continue to experience episodes in which their children's lives threatened with diarrhea in infancy – but they now know how to treat it, as few people would have known in the HICs' pre-transition period, and they have antibiotics available for managing severe cases where this is appropriate. Children in MICs do not enjoy a trouble-free childhood, but go through the distress of under-5 pneumonia or adolescent TB, while their parents experience the anxiety of trying to secure the antimicrobials needed to treat these conditions: for 5 million children with pneumonia in LMICs annually, their parents are unable to do this (Laxminarayan et al. 2016). The use of antimicrobials along with other readily transferable technologies sustain different underlying life course narratives in LMICs compared to those that typify HICs.

Underlying Causes

Without a basic understanding of the causal processes that characterize changes in population health and health inequalities, it is not possible to evaluate normative claims about the co-existence of narrowing global health inequalities and the within country widening health inequalities. Sampling changes in a given time period and presenting them as trends (or as trends that are causally linked – with the suggestion that health benefits are, as it were, transferred from the middle classes of HICs to the workers of LMICs) can misrepresent the broad causal picture as it unfolds.

The last 100 years, both globally and within country, constitute one period in a long-term process of *widening* social inequality in health. Broadly speaking, social inequality in health has risen ever since the Middle Ages (perhaps surprisingly), when nobles and peasants seem to have had similar life expectancies (Antonovsky 1967; Bengtsson and van Poppel 2011). The late 19th and early 20th century period – in which social inequalities in health narrowed within those countries that emerged as HICs – was an anomaly.

To relate the trends to transition theory, roughly speaking, we can say that pestilence and famine affect all social classes; as societies transition to agriculture, the wealthy still have surprisingly little protection from the infectious and hygienic diseases that characterize this stage of close co-habitation with animals and increased human crowding. This "agricultural transition" lowers life expectancy for individuals while increasing population size – a qualified form of "improvement" in population health. Urbanization and the initially slow but eventually rapid growth in economic productivity associated with it, by contrast, both raise the life expectancy of the population and increase its size. However, this improvement both for individuals and for populations benefits those of higher SES more than those of lower SES, opening up differences in life expectancy that persist and for the most part continue to grow.

The only period in which social inequalities in health narrowed for a time was the classic period of hygienic and sanitary reform at the end of the 19th and beginning of the 20th centuries – when initial steps to establish safety of the food supply, clean water, and sewage were taken in HICs (Soares 2007). At this point, the happy confluence of political change (increasingly wide suffrage), scientific development (the germ theory of disease), and growth in GDP contributed strongly to this narrowing.

The post-war growth of the welfare state, including systems of universal health coverage, by contrast, has at best slowed the growth of social inequality in health: it has not moved us in the direction of social equality in health (Sreenivasan 2007; Mackenbach 2012; Reid 2016). The better off get more out of the "fourth stage" of epidemiological transition by the differential benefit they derive from programs like universal health coverage. This is not to say that such programs do not promote social equality in health: it is plausible that the poor would have been left yet further behind without them (Reid 2016).

This sampling question is significant for the normative work that the development narrative is supposed to do. The narrative of local divergence (the almost-best-off falling a bit behind) and global convergence (the worst off catching up) relies on sampling HICs just after the one period in which inequalities narrowed (thereby excluding that narrowing) and sampling LMICs at a moment in history that includes the LMIC version of that era in which (in HICs) inequalities narrowed. The underlying dynamic is that as health improves, it improves more for the better off than the worse off, absent a period where we acted on the gains that could be made by providing the basic infrastructure of public health. The broad trend is the same globally and within country: it does not reflect a tradeoff in which we forgo goods for the already pretty-well-off and give them to the worse-off. On the contrary, as we saw in the previous section, we have taken a path to improving life expectancy in LMICs that seems likely not to lead to the same gains. The inference from a given period of narrowing to a broader pattern of a gap being closed is illicit.

Implications for Global AMR Policy

The narrative of catching up ignores longer-term trends and obscures differences in typical and various life courses that cause the life expectancy gains in LMICs. Waning antimicrobial effectiveness will reveal the different underlying causes of these gains.

Current approaches to addressing the role of social determinants of health (SDOH) in the impact of AMR, consistent with the model of global health that gave us the accelerated transition, is medicalized: medical technology transfer again takes the place of political development; inappropriate standards of evidence (the movement towards implementing evidence-based standards in development) direct efforts towards primary prevention and treatment and away from inter-sectoral cooperation on health-related primordial prevention. (See King, Chap. 19, this volume; Silva et al. 2020.) The WHO *Global Action Plan* (2015a) speaks, for example, of "effective prevention of infections transmitted through sex or drug injection as well as better sanitation, hand washing, and food and water safety" as "core components of infectious disease prevention," (§36) and "more widespread recognition of antimicrobial medicines as a public good … [being] needed in order to strengthen regulation of their distribution, quality, and use" (§41) to address inappropriate antimicrobial use, and the development of awareness and improved veterinary education to address the overuse of antimicrobials in agriculture.

Awareness and education are inadequate to address the struggles of LMICs to promote appropriate antimicrobial use. These countries often make do with half the tax revenues proportionate to GDP or national income that HICs expect: enforcement to tame diversion and over-the-counter sales of antibiotics or the for-profit healthcare sector (a substantial source of poor prescribing – Kuo et al. 2017; Haire, Chap. 3, this volume; Liverani et al., Chap. 5, this volume; Ho and Lee, Chap. 25, this volume) are not free. Neither can LMICs confront the globalized agricultural sector that moves agricultural practices that involve the overuse of antibiotics from the increasingly intolerant regulatory environments of HICs to their permissive regulatory environments. To confront this would in turn require an end to pressure from global supply chains serving HIC-consumers against environmental and labour regulation in LMICs (the justice dimensions of such dependencies are explored in the social connectionist model of Young 2006). Focusing innovation in anthelmintics, for example, on the needs of human beings vulnerable to parasites would change treatment possibilities (in accordance with the call of Shawa et al., Chap. 10, this volume), while reducing or eliminating agricultural use and improving health-related infrastructure – both of which involve political and economic change – would change the distribution of health benefits.

In addition, there is another global structural relationship in inequalities related to antimicrobial use, insofar as antimicrobials are a common or public good, as discussed elsewhere in this volume (Smith and Coast, Chap. 17, this volume; Giubilini and Savulescu, Chap. 9, this volume). LMICs cannot "catch up" in antimicrobial use because HICs are on track to use them up, for their own needs or in service of HIC-led policies that encourage antimicrobial use in LMICs instead of balanced development, high taxation and regulation, and democratic empowerment, the context in which conservative antimicrobial use can be implemented as policy.

The problem of effective regulation and orientation of the pharmaceutical industry towards population needs is not isolated to LMICs. Generic drug shortages in HICs contribute to AMR by driving inappropriate prescribing (Shoham et al. 2016), and every action plan on AMR highlights the failure of industry to invest in new antimicrobials, and not the problem that new antimicrobials, when found, continue to be marketed and deployed in ways that encourage non-beneficial and marginally beneficial use.

AMR and Widening Within-Country Social Inequality in Health

Antimicrobials played a role in the so-called "fourth stage" of epidemiological transition, in which life expectancy has been extended by effective prevention and treatment for cancer and heart disease, among other medical conditions. Insofar as progress in addressing these large sources of disease burden for HICs involves advanced surgical and other tertiary care techniques (in addition to dietary change and tobacco control), this fourth transition relies on antibiotics that make surgical and immune-system suppressing chemotherapeutics possible. Even in countries with universal, comprehensive health care without financial barriers to access (like Canada), innovations in tertiary care provide more benefit to the better-off than the worse-off (Starfield 2011; Asada and Kephart 2007)[5] – contributing to the return to growing social inequality in health despite universal health coverage in contemporary medical care.

At a superficial level, we could speculate that the development of AMR in HICs could undo a line of medical progress that has widened social inequalities in health. But there would be many opportunities for reassertion of the general pattern of the last several centuries, the pattern of the well-off capturing a greater share of benefits and experiencing a lower share of burdens. Moderating the use of antimicrobials to preserve their effectiveness calls on solidarity as a value (Holm and Ploug, Chap. 21, this volume); the implications of waning antimicrobial efficacy will put stress on this same value. For example, the tertiary care interventions of the fourth epidemiological stage are becoming increasingly expensive due to AMR (Smith and Coast 2013; Cosgrove 2006; Teillant et al. 2015). This will continue for some time as those interventions gradually take on an unfavourable intrinsic harm-benefit tradeoff for the individual patient directly involved. It is only at this last stage (where the

[5]This is thought to be because the worse-off face barriers to access that are both practical and social (e.g. geographical proximity and social capital that generates attention to the expression of need and referrals); when they do access care, they have fewer resources that would enable them to benefit from it, e.g. the social and income support to enable recovery; furthermore, the care is less suited to their needs, given that complex chronic conditions have a social gradient.

harm-benefit tradeoff shifts) that the loss of this technology would potentially narrow health inequalities by de-implementation of "fourth stage" interventions that have widened social inequalities in health. The effects of specialty and disease interest group advocacy in the intervening period may well result in even greater capture of the resources of the system for the better-off. The increasing cost of supportive care to maintain current surgical interventions while responding to AMR may also feed a political discourse around system sustainability that contributes to eroding the comprehensiveness and depth of universal healthcare coverage. Social inequalities in health could continue to widen as services for those with less voice are eroded to enable the higher cost of coping with AMR in the tertiary care sector that has served higher income persons well.

This is not just a HIC story. The Millennial Development Goals focused on child mortality and mortality of late adolescence/early adulthood (TB; the infectious and hygienic diseases), while the Sustainable Development Goals (SDG) on which the WHO embarked in 2015 focus on developing universal health coverage (UHC) and access to tertiary care – important for delivering the care necessary for chronic diseases and causes of midlife mortality that middle income countries are beginning to experience (WHO 2015b). The expected health transition from a higher burden of infectious and hygienic diseases to a higher burden of chronic, noncommunicable disease has informed this policy move. However, as we saw, MICs in particular are subject to the double burden of emerging chronic noncommunicable diseases alongside persistent infectious and hygienic diseases; they also experience a heavy burden from counter-transitions as new infectious and hygienic burdens arise (Cook and Dummer 2004; Santosa et al. 2014; Defo 2014). There is evidence that the prevalence of hospital-based resistant microbes is inversely associated with national income (Alvarez-Uria et al. 2016), suggesting that LMICs will also bear a heavier burden of hospital-based AMR than HICs, at the same time that they face a heavier burden of community-based resistant diseases. These new health systems will face the same kinds of political struggles about universality, depth, and sustainability that are in play in HICs (Norheim et al. 2014). Given the extent of economic inequalities within these countries, they will face these political struggles without the social solidarity that is somewhat protective of the breadth and depth of UHC in HICs. Indeed, some have speculated that AMR could entirely derail the SDG of UHC (Jasovský et al. 2016).

Conclusion

The debate between sufficientists and prioritarians on the one hand and egalitarians on the other turns on deep relationships between concerns about the formalism of interpersonal measures and (by contrast) the evident strength of the moral claim of the needs of the worse off. It is true that formal interpersonal measures can mask different underlying realities that would engage different concerns about justice (and other important values). Nonetheless, a fully developed picture of those underlying realities does not necessarily support the case for priority or sufficiency as goals – whether on normative grounds or on grounds of practicality. Perhaps putting the breaks on an underlying reality (the long term trend of growing social inequality in health) is not ultimately feasible: the role that antimicrobials have played in narrowing global health inequalities suggests as much.

The current narrowing of the global gap in life expectancy will not lead to the gap closing if there are fundamental barriers to narrowing the gap built into the path to the current achievement. What looks like a normatively satisfying narrowing of the gap is in reality a period in which a limited version of a familiar (and known to be temporary) reversal of a long term trend is playing out.

In the mid to late 20th century, it was thought that there was a limit to the long-term trend of growing health inequalities – perhaps a natural limit around 75, at which point the better-off would stop gaining life expectancy and then further gains would involve the worse-off (within and between countries) catching up. This has not come about: life expectancy at the top of the scale continues to advance and cautious observers no longer try to predict the upper limit. There is no known end to improvements in the upper limit figure, and so no natural limit to the growth of social inequality in health.

This growing gap is morally complex: Who can object to saving a life of a fellow citizen on the grounds that someone far away does not have access to the same treatment? But our failure to imagine the downside of some having access to lifesaving interventions in their 10th and 11th decades and beyond while others have their prospects for a long and healthy life compromised by social determinants is just that – a failure of imagination.

A century ago, social inequality in health meant that some buried half or more of their children before the age of 5 while others experienced this heartache less frequently. The moral concern we feel when learning of a gap in life expectancy between 40 and 70 is palpable; we are familiar with these narratives and the death of children is a tragedy for which children are not blamed. Social inequality in health now looks quite different. It may mean that some will enjoy long and active retirements approaching the length of their working lives, helping with grandchildren and greeting great-grandchildren, while others manage multiple morbidities related to chronic disease while in their later working lives, juggling this simultaneously with responsibilities to others – perhaps the mental health challenges faced by their children, the substance use entanglements of their partner, and the caregiving needs of their parents who are in turn suffering in their 70s from the cumulative effects of their own chronic conditions as the life narrative legacy of their exposure to the social determinants of ill health. These caregiving responsibilities lead to loss of mobility and skill upgrading, leading to missed work opportunities and, in a technology-driven economy, even loss of work – and so (in turn) to late-life poverty and death shortly after retirement (if retirement is an option at all).

Through the lens of literature, we can look back sympathetically at the concrete social shape that health inequalities took in earlier eras (with Dickens, for example); the form they are taking today are often presented in statistical terms and we have yet to develop a cultural narrative that explores the relations of domination and subordination and shapes the sense of intrinsic moral concern that might be raised by these differences. We are likely to think that individuals bear responsibility for these conditions (utilitarian reformers of the nineteenth century likewise thought those who were worse off responsible for their poor health). Who fundraises by running a race for the cure in their 60s and who is crowd-sourcing to raise money for their own cancer treatment (for travel and loss of work income if that treatment is covered under a universal health system, or for expensive therapeutics not covered in that universal system) – and what micro, meso, and macro relations of power are embodied here?

The *prima facie* moral plausibility of a prioritarian or sufficientist commitment is placed in question by a long-term trend towards a world in which the well-off enjoy a life expectancy – perhaps – double that of the worse-off. Suppose that the situation continued such that the person running for the cure in their 60s would become the centenarian running for the cure, and so on. How long would one remain a sufficientist? At what point would the gap become large enough that an appeal to sufficiency would ring hollow, and closing the gap would become a worthy moral commitment? If AMR makes the tertiary care that has continued the widening of the gap in the fourth stage of epidemiological transition even more expensive, at what cost and opportunity cost will we pursue the continuation of that trend or resist its reversal?

Globally, the response to AMR must move beyond lip service to the most minimal social determinants of health (sanitation and water) and engage with the political and economic process of redistributing resources and power so that governments and professional bodies can effectively regulate pharmaceutical production, distribution, and prescribing across the public and private sectors, and so that the global working class and those living with the legacy of colonization and resource theft (Wenar 2008) – whose housing conditions and social security currently preclude them from benefiting from the primordial prevention of infectious and hygienic disease that most residents of HICs have at this point enjoyed for most of the past century – can survive and even flourish despite the loss of the contribution of antimicrobials to the so-called accelerated epidemiological transition.

References

Alvarez-Uria, G., S. Gandra, and R. Laxminarayan. 2016. Poverty and prevalence of antimicrobial resistance in invasive isolates. *International Journal of Infectious Diseases* 52: 59–61.

Anderson, E. 1999. What is the point of equality? *Ethics* 109 (2): 287–337.

———. 2010. Justifying the capabilities approach to justice. In *Measuring justice: Primary goods and capabilities*, ed. H. Brighouse and I. Robeyns, 81–100. Cambridge: Cambridge University Press.

Antonovsky, A. 1967. Social class, life expectancy and overall mortality. *The Milbank Memorial Fund Quarterly* 45: 31–73.

Asada, Y., and G. Kephart. 2007. Equity in health services use and intensity of use in Canada. *BMC Health Services Research* 7: 41.

Bengtsson, T., and F. van Poppel. 2011. Socioeconomic inequalities in death from past to present: An introduction. *Explorations in Economic History* 48: 343–356.

Case, A., and A. Deaton. 2015. Rising morbidity and mortality in midlife among white non-Hispanic Americans in the 21st century. *Proceedings of the National Academy of Sciences* 112: 15078–15083.

Coast, R.D., and J. Smith. 2020. The economics of resistance through an economic lens. In *Ethics and drug resistance: Collective responsibility for global public health,* ed. E. Jamrozik and M. Selgelid, pp. 281–296. Cham: Springer.

Cook, I.G., and T.J. Dummer. 2004. Changing health in China: Re-evaluating the epidemiological transition model. *Health Policy* 67: 329–343.

Cosgrove, S.E. 2006. The relationship between antimicrobial resistance and patient outcomes: Mortality, length of hospital stay, and health care costs. *Clinical Infectious Diseases* 42 (Suppl 2): S82–S89.

Defo, B.K. 2014. Beyond the 'transition' frameworks: The cross-continuum of health, disease and mortality framework. *Global Health Action* 7: 24804.

Frenk, J., J.L. Bobadilla, C. Stern, T. Frejka, and R. Lozano. 1991. Elements for a theory of the health transition. *Health Transition Review*: 21–38.

Giubilini, A., and J. Savulescu. 2020. Moral responsibility and the justification of policies to preserve antimicrobial effectiveness. In *Ethics and drug resistance: Collective responsibility for global public health,* ed. E. Jamrozik and M. Selgelid, pp. 143–156. Cham: Springer.

Haire, B. 2020. Providing universal access while avoiding antiretroviral resistance: Ethical tensions in HIV treatment. In *Ethics and drug resistance: Collective responsibility for global public health,* ed. E. Jamrozik and M. Selgelid, pp. 37–54. Cham: Springer.

Harhay, M.O., J. Horton, and P.L. Olliaro. 2010. Epidemiology and control of human gastrointestinal parasites in children. *Expert Review of Anti-Infective Therapy* 8: 219–234.

Harper, S., N.B. King, S.C. Meersman, M.E. Reichman, N. Breen, and J. Lynch. 2010. Implicit value judgments in the measurement of health inequalities. *The Milbank Quarterly* 88: 4–29.

Ho, C.W., and T. Lee. 2020. Global governance of anti-microbial resistance: A legal and regulatory toolkit. In Ethics and drug resistance: Collective responsibility for global public health, ed. E. Jamrozik and M. Selgelid, pp. 403–422. Cham: Springer.

Holm, S. and T. Ploug. 2020. Solidarity and antimicrobial resistance. In *Ethics and drug resistance: Collective responsibility for global public health,* ed. E. Jamrozik and M. Selgelid, pp. 347–358. Cham: Springer.

Hu, Y., B.L. Ellis, Y.Y. Yiu, M.M. Miller, J.F. Urban, L.Z. Shi, and R.V. Aroian. 2013. An extensive comparison of the effect of anthelmintic classes on diverse nematodes. *PLoS One* 8: e70702.

Jamrozik, E., and M.J. Selgelid. 2020. Drug-resistant infection: Causes, consequences, and responses. In *Ethics and drug resistance: Collective responsibility for global public health,* ed. E. Jamrozik and M. Selgelid, pp. 3–18. Cham: Springer.

Jasovský, D., J. Littmann, A. Zorzet, and O. Cars. 2016. Antimicrobial resistance-a threat to the world's sustainable development. *Upsala Journal of Medical Sciences* 121: 159–164.

King, N.B. 2020. Technological fixes and antimicrobial resistance. In *Ethics and drug resistance: Collective responsibility for Global Public Health,* ed. E. Jamrozik and M. Selgelid, pp. 311–321. Cham: Springer

King, N.B., S. Harper, and M.E. Young. 2012. Use of relative and absolute effect measures in reporting health inequalities: Structured review. *BMJ* 345: e5774.

Kuo, S.C., S.M. Shih, L.Y. Hsieh, T.Y. Lauderdale, Y.C. Chen, C.A. Hsiung, and S.C. Chang. 2017. Antibiotic restriction policy paradoxically increased private drug consumptions outside Taiwan's national health insurance. *The Journal of Antimicrobial Chemotherapy* 72: 1544–1545.

Laxminarayan, R., D. Sridhar, M. Blaser, M. Wang, and M. Woolhouse. 2016. Achieving global targets for antimicrobial resistance. *Science* 353: 874–875.

Liverani, M., L. Hashiguchi, M. Khan, and R. Coker. 2020. Antimicrobial resistance and the private sector in Southeast Asia. In *Ethics and drug resistance: Collective responsibility for global public health,* ed. E. Jamrozik and M. Selgelid, pp. 78–87. Cham: Springer.

Mackenbach, J.P. 1996. The contribution of medical care to mortality decline: McKeown revisited. *Journal of Clinical Epidemiology* 49: 1207–1213.

———. 2012. The persistence of health inequalities in modern welfare states: The explanation of a paradox. *Social Science & Medicine* 75: 761–769.

———. 2015. Should we aim to reduce relative or absolute inequalities in mortality? *European Journal of Public Health* 25: 185.

Mackenbach, J.P., P. Martikainen, G. Menvielle, and R. de Gelder. 2016. The arithmetic of reducing relative and absolute inequalities in health: A theoretical analysis illustrated with European mortality data. *Journal of Epidemiology and Community Health* 70: 730–736.

MacPherson, D.W., B.D. Gushulak, W.B. Baine, S. Bala, P.O. Gubbins, P. Holtom, and M. Segarra-Newnham. 2009. Population mobility, globalization, and antimicrobial drug resistance. *Emerging Infectious Diseases* 15: 1727.

Marmot, M. 2015. *The health gap: The challenge of an unequal world.* London: Bloomsbury Publishing.

McKenna, M.L., S. McAtee, P.E. Bryan, R. Jeun, T. Ward, J. Kraus, M.E. Bottazzi, P.J. Hotez, C.C. Flowers, and R. Mejia. 2017. Human intestinal parasite burden and poor sanitation in rural Alabama. *American Journal of Tropical Medicine and Hygiene* 97 (5): 1623–1628.

Møller, H. 2010. Tuberculosis and colonialism: Current tales about tuberculosis and colonialism in Nunavut. *Journal of Aboriginal Health* 6: 38–48.

Norheim, O.F. et al. 2014. *Making fair choices on the path to universal health coverage.* World Health Organization. http://www.who.int/choice/documents/making_fair_choices/en/. Accessed 15 Sept 2017.

Nussbaum, M.C. 2006. *Frontiers of justice: Disability, nationality, species membership.* Cambridge, MA: Harvard University Press.

O'Neill, J. 2014. *Antimicrobial resistance: Tackling a crisis for the health and wealth of nations.* https://amr-review.org/sites/default/files/AMR%20Review%20Paper%20-%20Tackling%20a%20crisis%20for%20the%20health%20and%20wealth%20of%20nations_1.pdf. Accessed 15 Sept 2017.

Olshansky, S.J., and A.B. Ault. 1986. The fourth stage of the epidemiologic transition: The age of delayed degenerative diseases. *The Milbank Quarterly* 64 (3): 355–391.

Omran, A.R. 1971. The epidemiologic transition: A theory of the epidemiology of population change. *The Milbank Memorial Fund Quarterly* 4 (1): 509–538.

O'Neill, J. 2016. *Review on antimicrobial resistance.* https://amr-review.org/sites/default/files/160525_Final%20paper_with%20cover.pdf. Accessed 15 Sept 2017.

Orr, P. 2013. Tuberculosis in Nunavut: Looking back, moving forward. *CMAJ* 185: 287–288.

Parfit, D. 1997. Equality and priority. *Ratio* 10: 202–221.

———. 2012. Another defence of the priority view. *Utilitas* 24: 399–440.

Piketty, T. 2014. *Capital in the twenty-first century.* Cambridge, MA: Harvard University Press.

Pilkington, E. 2017. Hookworm, a disease of extreme poverty, is thriving in the US south. Why? *The Guardian*, https://www.theguardian.com/us-news/2017/sep/05/hookworm-lowndes-county-alabama-water-waste-treatment-poverty.

Regidor, E. 2004. Measures of health inequalities: Part 2. *Journal of Epidemiology and Community Health* 58: 900–903.

Reid, L. 2016. Answering the empirical challenge to arguments for universal health coverage based in health equity. *Public Health Ethics* 9: 231–243.

Santosa, A., S. Wall, E. Fottrell, U. Högberg, and P. Byass. 2014. The development and experience of epidemiological transition theory over four decades: A systematic review. *Global Health Action* 7: 59–71.

Sen, A. 2002. Why health equity? *Health Economics* 11: 659–666.

Shawa, R., F. Coomans, H. Cox, and L. London. 2020. Access to effective treatment for drug resistant tuberculosis: Deepening the human rights-based approach. In *Ethics and drug resistance: Collective responsibility for global public health*, ed. E. Jamrozik and M. Selgelid, pp. 157–171. Cham: Springer.

Shoham, S., A.A. Antar, P.G. Auwaerter, C.M. Durand, M.S. Sulkowski, and D.J. Cotton. 2016. Antimicrobial access in the 21st century: Delays and critical shortages. *Annals of Internal Medicine* 165: 53–54.

Silva, J., A.M. Viens, and D.S. Littmann. 2020. The super-wicked problem of antimicrobial resistance. In *Ethics and drug resistance: Collective responsibility for global public health*, ed. E. Jamrozik and M. Selgelid, pp. 423–445. Cham: Springer.

Smith, R., and J. Coast. 2013. The true cost of antimicrobial resistance. *BMJ* 346: f1493–f1493.

Soares, R.R. 2007. On the determinants of mortality reductions in the developing world. *Population and Development Review* 33: 247–287.

Sreenivasan, G. 2007. Health care and equality of opportunity. *The Hastings Center Report* 37: 21–31.

Starfield, B. 2011. The hidden inequity in health care. *International Journal for Equity in Health* 10: 15.

Strømme, E.M., and O.F. Norheim. 2017. Global health inequality: Comparing inequality-adjusted life expectancy over time. *Public Health Ethics* 10: 188–211.

Suk, J.E., D. Manissero, G. Büscher, and J.C. Semenza. 2009. Wealth inequality and tuberculosis elimination in Europe. *Emerging Infectious Diseases* 15: 1812–1814.

Teillant, A., S. Gandra, D. Barter, D.J. Morgan, and R. Laxminarayan. 2015. Potential burden of antibiotic resistance on surgery and cancer chemotherapy antibiotic prophylaxis in the USA: A literature review and modelling study. *The Lancet Infectious Diseases* 15: 1429–1437.

Temkin, L.S. 2000. Equality, priority, and the levelling down objection. In *The ideal of equality*, ed. M. Clayton and A. Williams, 126–161. Basingstoke: Macmillan.

———. 2003. Egalitarianism defended. *Ethics* 113: 764–782.

Valles, S.A. 2018. *Philosophy of population health science: Philosophy for a new public health era*. London/New York: Routledge/Taylor & Francis Group.

Venkatapuram, S., and M. Marmot. 2013. *Health justice an argument from the capabilities approach*. New York: Wiley.

Walzer, M. 2008. *Spheres of justice: A defense of pluralism and equality*. New York: Basic Books.

Wenar, L. 2008. Property rights and the resource curse. *Philosophy & Public Affairs* 36: 2–32.

Wolff, J., and A. da Shalit. 2007. *Disadvantage*. Oxford: Oxford University Press.

World Health Organization (WHO). 2015a. *Global action plan on antimicrobial resistance*. http://www.who.int/antimicrobial-resistance/publications/global-action-plan/en/. Accessed 13 Dec 2018.

———. 2015b. *Health in 2015: from Millennium Development Goals (MDG) to Sustainable Development Goals (SDG)*. https://www.who.int/gho/publications/mdgs-sdgs/en/. Accessed 13 Dec 2018.

Young, I.M. 2006. Responsibility and global justice: A social connection model. *Social Philosophy and Policy* 23: 102–130.

3

A Capability Perspective on Antibiotic Resistance, Inequality, and Child Development

Michael Millar

Abstract Nussbaum's capability theory by drawing attention to multiple determinants of wellbeing provides a rich and relevant evaluative space for framing antibiotic resistance. I consider the implications of antibiotic resistance for child development and adult capabilities. There are common risk factors for childhood growth stunting and the spread of infectious diseases in both antibiotic sensitive and resistant forms. The interaction between infectious diseases, antibiotic resistance and growth stunting illustrates a clustering of disadvantage. The control of antibiotic resistance requires wide-ranging cooperative action. Cooperation is predicated on an expectation of equitable access to effective antibiotics. This expectation is confounded by inequality both in access to antibiotics, and in the risk that available antibiotics will be ineffective. Securing child development (and adult capabilities) requires that inequalities both in access to antibiotics and in risk factors for the dissemination and transmission of antibiotic resistance are addressed. Inequality undermines the cooperative activity that is control of infectious diseases and compounds the threat to the securing of capabilities that arises from antibiotic resistance.

Keywords Antibiotics · Capabilities and growth stunting · Social justice · Mother and child health · Infectious Disease

Introduction

Antibiotic resistance has been framed as a problem consequent on the lack of development of new antibiotics and overuse of existing antibiotics. How we frame a problem is important in determining our responses to the problem (Tversky and Kahneman 1981). Unsurprisingly solutions to antibiotic resistance have been

M. Millar (✉)
Barts Health NHS Trust, London, UK
e-mail: M.R.Millar@qmul.ac.uk

focused on developing new antibiotics, and constraining the use of existing antibiotics (see for example http://drive-ab.eu, and https://www.bu.edu/law/faculty-scholarship/carb-x). Yet, new antibiotics and constraints on use of existing antibiotics can never be a solution to the potentiation of infectious disease transmission (in antibiotic sensitive or resistant forms) consequent on poverty, over-crowding, malnutrition, limited educational opportunity, environmental degradation, poor water quality, inadequate sanitation or conflict.

Capability Theory

Capability theory has been influential in defining measures of human development, and quality of life, and in the evaluation of the justice of social arrangements. Sen (1999) defined a capability as a 'substantial freedom he or she enjoys to lead the kind of life he or she has reason to value'. Nussbaum emphasises the importance of capabilities for human dignity, and derives entitlements from reflecting on the requirements for equal dignity and respect. She describes necessary conditions for a decently just society, in the form of a set of ten fundamental entitlements for all citizens (Nussbaum 2006). More recently capability theory has been applied to children (Biggeri et al. 2011) and child development (Peleg 2013). Nussbaum and Dixon (2012) have proposed that capability theory can be used to provide theoretical justification, and to justify a degree of special state priority for children's rights – based on the 'unique vulnerability of children to the decisions of others' (Nussbaum and Dixon 2012, p. 575).

Antibiotic resistance has implications for child development, basic capabilities, and the securing of adult capabilities. There is on-going debate about the elements that should be included in a capabilities list that is appropriate for adults (Wolff and De-Shalit 2007) or children (Biggeri and Mehrotra 2011). Children develop in to adults, moving through different developmental stages and capabilities at different ages. Child development both depends on the capabilities of adult carers, and determines the potential for adult capabilities. For the purposes of this chapter I have accepted the list that Nussbaum proposes as appropriate for adults, and that achievement of thresholds of adult capabilities is substantially dependent on child development. The capabilities listed by Nussbaum (2006, p. 154) encompass life expectancy, bodily health & integrity, sense, imagination and thought, emotions, practical reason, affiliation, relations with other species, play and control over one's environment.

Infectious Disease and Capabilities

The use of antibiotics can be conceptualised as an attempt to try to prevent damage caused by infection to established capabilities (adults) or the potential for capabilities (children). One consequence of the use of antibiotics is antibiotic resistance.

The rate at which antibiotic resistance develops is a function of usage, time, control measures, and the context of use. The availability of effective treatments for infectious disease is a substantial determinant of health. The interactions between health and the determinants of health are complex and not unidirectional, so for example health both determines and is determined by nutrition, education, and social status. The extent of capability fulfilment can be used to define health, while health is required for the fulfilment of capabilities (Venkatapuran 2011, 2013). Uncontrolled infectious disease subverts the achievement of adult capabilities through multiple pathways including through damage to child development. Damage to the capabilities of adult carers also has consequences for child development.

The control of infectious diseases (antibiotic sensitive and resistant) requires fulfilment of multiple entitlements. An entitlement to bodily health requires that an individual is able to have good health, including reproductive health; to be adequately nourished; and to have adequate shelter. The adequacy of shelter is important as a risk factor for the spread of infectious disease, and for damage to child development (see for example Shelter 2006). Nutrition influences both child development and infectious disease susceptibility (Gough et al. 2014). Maternal reproductive health is an important determinant of child development and vulnerability to infectious disease. A capability for senses, imagination, and thought requires education. To secure child development we must secure the capabilities of those who care for them. Nussbaum and Dixon (2012) emphasise that 'the goal remains the full empowerment of all individuals' (p. 578). Maternal education is a key element in assuring healthy child development (see discussion of growth stunting below). Maternal education and parental control of their local environment are necessary elements in protecting children from infectious disease. The entitlements to be able to play and to have relationships with the world of nature can be qualified by adding 'safely'. Children in developing countries may not be able to live and play without exposure to the risk of infectious diseases (antibiotic sensitive and resistant) transmitted as a result of poor sanitation, close proximity to animals with zoonotic infection, and vectors for disease (such as malaria mosquitoes). Infectious disease contributes to impairment of child development through multiple pathways including growth stunting (discussed further below).

The capabilities listed by Nussbaum remind us of important dimensions of the individual experience of infectious disease (such as freedom of movement and engagement in social interactions). The entitlement to affiliation requires that an individual is able to live for and in relation to others, to recognize and show concern for other human beings, and to engage in various forms of social interaction. Bodily integrity requires that an individual can move freely from place to place. These last two entitlements can be breached by restrictions taken to control the spread of infectious disease (antibiotic sensitive or resistant), and by the social consequences of infectious disease, particularly when associated with treatment (antibiotic) resistance (see for example Upshur et al. 2009).

Constraints on freedoms to prescribe, to purchase, to manufacture and formulate, to dispose, to pollute, and to use antibiotics for economic gain can all contribute to the control of antibiotic resistance. Nussbaum's approach does not preclude limitations on freedoms with respect to the use of antibiotics. Nussbaum gives emphasis to the need to limit freedoms when those freedoms adversely impact on the central capabilities. She states that 'no society that pursues equality or even an ample social minimum can avoid curtailing freedom in very many ways, and what it ought to say is those freedoms are not good, they are not part of a core group of entitlements required by the notion of social justice, and in many ways, indeed, they may subvert those core entitlements' (Nussbaum 2011, p. 73). 'In other words, all societies that pursue a reasonably just political conception have to evaluate human freedoms, saying that some are central and some trivial, some good and some actively bad, some deserving of special protection and others not' (Nussbaum 2011, pp. 74–75). Framing the actions, constraints and precautions from a capability perspective also identifies limits to the precautions that we can take and gives priority to actions, which do not undermine capability entitlements. A policy that results in a substantial loss of a capability for some can be challenged from a capability perspective, even if there was an overall benefit. Stigmatisation, isolation, and segregation of individuals to prevent the spread of treatment resistant infection (such as leprosy historically) would not be consistent with a capability perspective while there remain feasible alternative courses of action. The non-availability of effective treatments resulting from antibiotic resistance restricts alternative courses of action. For much of the twentieth century women with leprosy were actively discouraged or prevented from having children. New-born babies of mothers with leprosy were taken from their parents at birth, because otherwise the child would also develop leprosy (see for example International Leprosy Association, History of Leprosy). Capabilities related to childbirth including the opportunities to have and to look after a child were removed. Leprosy has now been controlled to a large extent by the advent and availability of effective antibiotic treatments.

Human Dignity and Infectious Disease

An emphasis on thc importance of human dignity is a substantial element within Nussbaum's capability theory. There is a lack of consensus on how best to define and measure human dignity (Ashcroft 2005). Dignity can be defined positively but also negatively as freedom from sources of humiliation (see Shultziner and Rabinovici 2011). Nussbaum, while acknowledging that dignity is a poorly defined concept, uses human dignity as a touchstone for the selection of capabilities. Nussbaum's list of capabilities is a list of positive entitlements (capabilities) that are necessary for the living of a life with human dignity. Respect for the dignity of others is an important social and political value. Conditions must pertain that reflect that value and these include conditions that foster a sense of personal worth in each person.

There are strong associations between social status, self-esteem and health (Mann 1998; Marmot 2003; Chilton 2006). There are many ways in which dignity interacts with infectious diseases. There are common risk factors for violations of dignity and infectious diseases, for example lack of access to safe toilets contributes to loss of dignity, gender-based violence, and the transmission of infectious disease (see WHO factsheet 392). Inadequate shelter threatens dignity and increases infectious disease risks (Shelter 2006). Some infectious diseases, particularly those that are difficult to treat, such as antibiotic resistant tuberculosis, increase the risk that the dignity of adults will be violated (Upshur et al. 2009). Children with HIV or with a parent with HIV can suffer a substantial loss of self-esteem (Chi and Li 2014). An individual or group with an infectious disease may suffer from stigmatisation, social isolation, and a resultant loss of a sense of self-worth. Social consequences of infection for individuals, groups and institutions also include blame and shame (Sontag 1989). Acquisition and carriage of antibiotic resistant bacteria by individuals while undergoing healthcare can be associated with stigmatisation (Rump et al. 2017). Public health policies designed to support the control of antibiotic resistant bacteria can also lead to stigmatisation of individuals (Ploug et al. 2015). Violations of dignity and damage to self-esteem can increase infectious disease risk through changes in human behaviour. Low self-esteem is associated with sexual risk taking behaviour and sexually transmitted disease (see Byrnes et al. 1999; Ethier et al. 2006).

There are common risk factors for violations of dignity and infectious diseases, violations of dignity increase infectious disease risk, and infectious disease increases the risk that dignity will be violated.

Clustering of Disadvantage: The Example of Growth Stunting

In discussing actions which lead to the destruction of capabilities Nussbaum states that ‘We can certainly agree that capability-destruction in children is a particularly grave matter and as such should be off-limits’. ‘Usually situations are not so grave, and thus in many such cases the approach has little to say, allowing matters to be settled through the political process’ (Nussbaum 2011, p. 27). Unfortunately capability-destruction is not unusual in many countries. It is estimated that more than 40% of children in lower and middle income countries are at risk of impaired development (Black et al. 2016). A period of particular risk to development is that between conception and 3 years of age. More than 25% of children <5 years of age globally have stunted growth (low height-for-age). Stunting is associated with long-term cognitive and physical impairment (Hair et al. 2015; Noble et al. 2015) and substantial economic consequences for individuals, communities and countries (Horton and Steckel 2013). The WHO Conceptual Framework for stunted growth (Stewart et al. 2013) identifies a range of community and societal contextual factors underlying the causes of stunting of growth of children. These factors include political arrangements, poverty, regulatory frameworks, healthcare systems, beliefs and norms, the status of women, access to safe foods, sanitation, population density, and natural and manmade disasters. Solutions require intervention in multiple sectors with specific emphasis given to the way in which resources are controlled and distributed through the political and economic system, food security, education (particularly of females), water quality, sanitation (and hygiene), ameliorating poverty and vulnerability, and access to healthcare (Casanovas et al. 2013). Nussbaum's capability approach specifies a broad range of entitlements and in so doing is well placed to explicitly accommodate these multiple and complex requirements.

Infections are thought to contribute to the pathogenesis of growth stunting and infections are both more common and more serious in children with stunting. Recently it has been suggested that administration of antibiotics to populations of children could be used to prevent stunted growth (Gough et al. 2014). The proposal to use antibiotics as a population level intervention to mitigate the risk of stunting illustrates the tension between sustaining effective antibiotics while assuring access for those in pressing need. Population level antibiotic interventions have profound implications for present and future generations particularly when the target populations live under conditions of relative deprivation that facilitate the spread of agents of infection in sensitive and resistant forms. Common risk factors for stunting and for the spread of infectious diseases include overcrowding, poor education (particularly maternal), poor nutrition, inadequate sanitation, and poor water quality. Capability insufficiencies (such as poor shelter, threats to bodily health, lack of access to maternal education) contribute both to the transmission of infectious disease and to host susceptibility to disease, and potentially to the burden of antibiotic resistance. There is a clustering of disadvantage in that infectious disease amplifies other disadvantages consequent on capability insufficiencies.

The use of antibiotics in many developed economies has extended beyond the treatment and prevention of life-threatening human infections to include the mitigation of symptoms of self-limiting disease(s), animal husbandry, fish farming, and to allow us to extend the range of medical and surgical interventions including those with limited health benefits such as some forms of cosmetic surgery. In developed countries antibiotics have become a means to a variety of ends, with varying degrees of relationship with mitigation of harm to human capabilities. Despite this there is evidence that the use of antibiotics in developed countries has stabilised or fallen this century (van Boeckel et al. 2014). Most of the recent increase in use of antibiotics has been in rapidly developing countries including Brazil, Russia, India, China and South Africa (BRICS countries). Holland particularly has shown how it is possible for developed countries to have low levels of human antibiotic usage and low levels of antibiotic resistance associated with patients (http://www.ecdc.europa.eu/en/activities/surveillance/EARS-Net/Pages/Index.aspx). By contrast antibiotic resistance is more prevalent now in developing countries with high levels of deprivation than in developed countries (WHO Report 2014). This situation probably reflects the capacity of countries to expend resources on trying to assure socio-economic conditions (and capability entitlements) such as education, health, nutrition, sanitation, and housing which are significant determinants of the epidemiology of infectious disease. An oft-quoted example of this relationship is that of tuberculosis. The incidence of tuberculosis (TB) and the requirement to treat TB has declined dramatically over recent decades in developed countries and this decline has been attributed to improvements in socio-economic conditions (Comstock 2000). By contrast with developed countries such as Holland the context of use of antibiotics in low to middle income countries frequently involves heightened conditions for the spread of infectious diseases both in antibiotic sensitive and resistant forms.

Antibiotic resistance considered from within a capability perspective draws attention to the importance of the social, political and economic context in determining infectious disease risks. Antibiotic resistance threatens to place an additional burden on communities where growth stunting and infection are already prevalent, because many of the risk factors for growth stunting also determine the risk that antibiotic resistance will spread. Capabilities may be incommensurable but capabilities still interact with each other in contributing to a state of wellbeing. In the real world these interactions may lead to clustering of disadvantage (Wolff and De-Shalit 2007). The interaction of infection with growth stunting in children illustrates the clustering of disadvantage and the importance of addressing the broad range of capability deficiencies. Otherwise preventable childhood stunting has the potential to persist alongside burgeoning levels of antibiotic resistance.

Capability Thresholds and Inequality?

'The basic claim of my account of social justice is this: respect for human dignity requires that citizens be placed above an ample threshold of capability in all ten of those areas' (Nussbaum 2011, p. 36). In this section I ask if capability thresholds can be achieved while there remains avoidable and substantial inequality in access to effective antibiotics and in the determinants of infectious disease. Inequality can be and often is harmful to human wellbeing (Picket and Wilkinson 2010). Our sense of self-worth, our social status, our wellbeing and inequalities are intertwined (Marmot 2003, 2005). Thresholds of capability may not achievable while substantial inequalities remain. Wolff and De-Shalit (2007, p. 10) define a society of equals as one in which 'disadvantages do not cluster, where there is no clear answer to the question of who is the worst off'. Certainly countries are not equal partners and neither are individuals within countries, when account is taken of the burdens of infectious disease – as exemplified by the contrasting patterns of child development and the clustering of disadvantage.

There is inequality in access to effective antibiotics (Laxminarayan et al. 2016). Pneumonia is still responsible for 1 in 5 deaths of children less than five years old in the world today. Ensuring access of children with pneumonia to antibiotics has been a major objective of the WHO and UNICEF over the last decade (WHO 2013). There is also inequality in the risk of acquisition of antibiotic resistant bacteria. There is increasing evidence of extensive environmental contamination with antibiotics and antibiotic resistant bacteria (Lubbert et al. 2017), particularly from antibiotic manufacturing plants, from use of antibiotics in meat production, from hospitals and urban conurbations (Berendonk et al. 2015). There is increasing use of antibiotics to support animal meat production even in countries with high levels of childhood growth stunting (see Centre for Science and Environment Report 2014). It is estimated that by 2030 the use of antibiotics in livestock production in the US and China will account for 40% of global antibiotic use (Van Boeckel et al. 2015). Antibiotic resistant bacteria, selected in humans and animals, are shared through environmental pollution with both those who can and those who cannot afford to eat meat. Often those with less or no access to antibiotics live in conditions, which promote the spread of antibiotic resistance. These differences are particularly strong in countries where some live in relative affluence in close proximity to slums. Those who are better off have access to the best medical advice, diagnostics for antibiotic resistance, and the latest treatments including antibiotics. When antibiotic resistant bacteria contaminate the environment of people with inadequate sanitation, poor education and with a heightened susceptibility to disease then spread is facilitated. Contamination of the Ganges provides a specific example. While the rich can afford cremation on the Ganges, and pilgrimage to the upper Ganges, the poor cannot. The water of the Ganges has become highly polluted with antibiotic resistant bacteria including a particularly worrying form of antibiotic resistance called New Delhi Metallo-β-lactamase (NDM-1) (Ahammad et al. 2014). Poor people use the water of the Ganges for recreation, washing, and drinking. Poor people with limited access to medical care or antibiotics are exposed to extreme forms of antibiotic resistance through day-to-day activities, with implications for the efficacy of antibiotics, their health and for the health of those around them. There is inequality in the risk of acquisition of antibiotic resistance as well as inequality in access to effective antibiotics (see Note 1).

International Cooperation, Unequal Partners

Currently the majority of countries collaborate on the control of infectious diseases. One hundred and ninety-six countries have signed up to the International Health Regulations (2005) (developed after the SARS outbreak in 2003), which are designed to control the international spread of infectious disease. The control of epidemic diseases is included in the United Nations Rights Document A/6316 (1996). Over recent years antibiotic resistance has become a focus of international concern. The World Health Organisation (2015) has developed an action plan for antimicrobial resistance, which recognises the need for international collaboration (for example see Section 21 (4), Global Action Plan). There is also broad acceptance in the scientific literature (see for example Institute of Medicine 2010) that control of antibiotic resistance requires international cooperative action.

Unequal relationships between countries can subvert cooperation. For example Indonesia has had outbreaks of avian influenza, which have been associated with high mortality, yet withdrew from cooperation with the WHO Global Influenza Surveillance Network (GISN) in 2007. The position from the Indonesian perspective is described in a journal article as follows – 'Indonesia believes that the world must work in unity against the H5N1 virus infection.... The work must be conducted side by side with mutual trust, transparency and equity as global citizens professionals, taking into consideration the elements of human dignity and solidarity.' 'The avian influenza case in Indonesia has demonstrated once again the unresolved imbalance between the affluent 'high-tech' countries and poor agriculture-based countries. Countries that are the hardest hit by a disease must also bear the burden of the cost of the vaccine, therapeutics and other products, while the monetary and non-monetary benefits of these products go to the manufacturers that are mostly in the industrialised countries' (Sedyaningsih et al. 2008, p. 487). Indonesia and other resource poor countries were expected to participate in cooperating in the control of infectious disease, yet there was a belief that the benefits of cooperation were unequally distributed. Subsequently an agreement was reached which stipulated arrangements for more equitable cooperative arrangements (World Health Assembly 2011).

Another example of an unequal international relationship that relates more directly to the control of antibiotic resistance arises from the Kumarasamy et al. report in 2010 that New Delhi Metallo-β-lactamase-1 was widespread in India. The Indian government considered this name to be 'unfair' and stigmatising, and potentially undermined the burgeoning health tourist market in India (see Pandey 2010). The Editor of the Lancet subsequently described the use of this name as an error and apologized stating that the name had 'unnecessarily stigmatised a single country and city' (Sinhal 2011). This interaction has compromised research on the epidemiology of NDM-1 in India according to the lead author of the Lancet report (Tim Walsh), who named this form of resistance NDM-1. He stated that 'We were banned from India and India had a massive clampdown on sending (biological) strains out' (Sugden 2013). Health tourism is developing fast in India and the stigma associated with the potential acquisition of antibiotic resistant bacteria was characterised by Indian politicians as an international plot to undermine that development. Unfortunately NDM1 is now globally distributed (Berrazeg et al. 2014). Conflict between the Lancet and the Indian government over health policy has continued (Sinhal 2015).

This second story illustrates aspects of the epidemiology of antibiotic resistance. When social conditions are poor then antibiotics quickly become ineffective, antibiotic resistant bacteria can be rapidly spread around the world, and there is a relationship between the sustaining of the functions of antibiotics and other socio-economic 'goods' such as adequate shelter, and clean water. This example also illustrates a relationship between antibiotic resistance, and stigma, which can undermine cooperation in the control of antibiotic resistance. There is considerable inequality in the international influence of the biomedical press with a bias towards developed countries with a strong research base. Combinations of economic inequality, antibiotic prescribing practice norms, and publication practice have marked out India in a way that adds additional disadvantage in a competitive global market for medical tourism.

A Relational Approach to Capability Inequality

Nussbaum argues that a contractualist account (such as that proposed by Scanlon 1998) based on individuals as moral equals 'is a powerful intuitive way of capturing the idea that human beings are moral equals despite their widely differing circumstances in an unequal world' (Nussbaum 2006, p. 272). Nussbaum states that 'I employ the notion of reasonable rejection, or something very close to it, in articulating my account of political justification' (Nussbaum 2011, p. 89). Her approach 'is a partial account of specifically political entitlements' (Nussbaum 2011, p. 96).

Scanlon provides an account of why and when we can reject both distributive and non-distributive inequalities (see Scanlon 2003, 2013) which can be applied to Nussbaum's evaluative capability framework. Reasonable rejection and justification to others provide the substantial focus of Scanlon's contractualist approach (Scanlon 1998) (for more discussion of Scanlon's approach see Note 2). Interactions between individuals and groups determine the epidemiology of infectious diseases. Human relations directly or indirectly have a substantial role in the spread of infectious diseases. In addition many of the transactions that determine the use of antibiotics and the consequences of use involve individuals, institutions and nations in dialogue. Examples include healthcare workers (such as doctors) agreeing treatment plans with patients, or healthcare authorities and institutions agreeing antibiotic policies within nations, or nations agreeing approaches to international collaboration on the control of antibiotic resistance. Justification is a key element to these relational interactions and it seems intuitively attractive to start from an acknowledgement of the importance of justification in assuring the validity of principles and agreements. Another attractive feature of Scanlon's approach is a concern with assuring the conditions for self-worth. This is significant both in relation to the epidemiology of infectious disease (as previously discussed) and in relation to a concern with assuring the conditions for a life with human dignity (a substantial concern for Nussbaum's capability theory) (Fitzpatrick 2008).

For Scanlon everyone counts morally, regardless of race, gender, or where they live. The different reasons for rejecting inequalities are dependent 'on the way that an inequality affects or arises from the relations between individuals' (see Scanlon lecture – Why does inequality matter?). Reasons for rejecting inequalities 'presuppose some form of relationship or interaction between unequal parties' and are based on comparing the differences in the situations of individuals (Scanlon (2004) lecture – When does equality matter?). For Scanlon (2006) reasonable rejection does not depend on rejection of the distribution of goods, but rather it depends on assuring equal respect and fairness. Nussbaum's capability theory provides an evaluative framework for the extent to which equal respect and fairness are achieved, without being itself a complete theory of distributive justice.

Scanlon argues that 'relief of suffering, avoidance of stigmatising differences in status, prevention of domination by others, and the preservation of conditions of procedural fairness are basic and important moral values' (Scanlon 2003, p. 218) that can give reason to reject inequalities. Inequalities can also be rejected when there are institutional obligations to provide certain benefits in an even-handed way, or 'cases in which individuals, as participants in a cooperative endeavour, have at least a *prima facie* claim to an equal share of the goods which that endeavour produces' (Scanlon 2013, p. 463). The control of antibiotic resistance is a cooperative exercise. Cooperation is predicated on an expectation of a share in access to effective antibiotics. Importantly the scope of these reasons for rejection of inequalities extends beyond national boundaries (for a fuller discussion see O'Neill 2013).

Inequalities Subvert Capabilities

Inequalities can lead to substantial disadvantage, furthering inequalities in a competitive world, and cluster to give multiple disadvantages. Inequalities can result in stigmatising differences in status, both at the level of the individual and the state as shown by the example of NDM-1 antibiotic resistance described above. Inequalities in access to antibiotics coexist with inequalities in risk factors for infection, and risk factors for antibiotic resistance. These inequalities can and do contribute to social, political and economic disadvantage, as exemplified by the interactions between childhood growth stunting, infectious diseases and antibiotic access.

Wealth determines access to healthcare, medicines (including antibiotics) and healthy living conditions. The less wealthy in many countries have less access to high quality medicines, little access to medical advice, or diagnostic facilities, often live under conditions that may facilitate the spread of antibiotic resistant bacteria, may be exposed to resistant bacteria even before exposure to antibiotics, and are more at risk of infection, and of the serious consequences from infection. Securing child development requires control of infectious diseases in treatment sensitive and resistant forms. There is an unequal distribution of childhood burdens and benefits associated with antibiotics and antibiotic resistance both within and between countries. These inequalities contribute to avoidable suffering (preventable infectious disease), differences in status (growth stunting), and potentially domination of vulnerable children by others. Inequalities subvert the achievement of capability thresholds.

Addressing Inequalities, AchievingCapability Thresholds

Control of antibiotic resistance is a cooperative enterprise with shared objectives and shared responsibilities. Countries cooperate in the control of infectious disease including antibiotic-resistant agents of infection. If we accept that all of the parties engaged in the control of antibiotic resistance should have an equal *prima facie* claim to access to effective antibiotics then when inequalities exist we can ask if those inequalities can be justified – 'basic structures need to be justified to all who are asked to accept them' (Scanlon lecture – Why Does Inequality Matter?) (see Note 3).

Developed countries have used antibiotics for much longer and in much larger quantities and for a wider range of reasons than most developing nations. India is subject to criticism for insufficient regulation of antibiotic prescribing. Yet, even by 2010, India used half the number of antibiotic units per person compared with the USA (Laxminarayan and Chaudhury 2016). Historically while new antibiotics were regularly coming to the market there was no commercial motivation to constrain antibiotic use because antibiotic resistance was a major justification for using the new antibiotic(s). The profits from antibiotic sales were largely accrued by companies based in the developed world. Marketing decisions were dominated by consideration of profit maximisation with a relatively low priority given to public health. The United Nations has accepted that developed nations should take up a greater part of the responsibility for the control of greenhouse gases than developing countries. 'Common but Differentiated Responsibilities' (UNFCCC 2015) are justified because there are differences in capacity to respond, different priorities, and differences in the historical contribution to the problem of greenhouse gas emissions between developed and developing countries. These differences also apply to antibiotic resistance.

In the World Health Assembly Global Action Plan for Antimicrobial Resistance (2015) Section 21. (3) **Access** states that '*The aim to preserve the ability to treat serious infections requires both equitable access to, and appropriate use of, existing and new antimicrobial medicines*'. Currently despite the high level of international concern there is no international agreement as to what constitutes 'appropriate' use of antibiotics. Equitable access is a long way away when account is taken of the lack of access to antibiotics for the treatment of life-threatening infection in many parts of the world while antibiotics are used extensively without human health benefit in many other parts of the world. I have previously argued that appropriate use is that which prevents some substantial risk of irretrievable harm in patients or their contacts, where a substantial risk is a level of risk which exceeds the range of risks of irretrievable harm that we tolerate in our day to day lives (Millar 2012). Use of antibiotics to support (non-human) animal growth promotion is inappropriate use. Use of antibiotics for animal growth promotion has been reported to be increasing in both developed and developing countries (Van Boeckel et al. 2015), including in areas where human growth stunting is particularly prevalent such as Sub-Saharan Africa. In developing countries people are more likely to live in close proximity to animals, so that the risks that antibiotic resistant bacteria will spread from animals, and that people will be exposed to antibiotics present in their environment, is increased compared with developed countries where the close proximity of farm animals with people is less common. It is strikingly inappropriate for many children to have limited access to antibiotics while antibiotics are being used as animal growth promoters. Developed countries should take a lead in limiting use of antibiotics as animal growth promoters.

The UN has given a substantial place to human dignity in the Sustainable Development Goals (UN 2014). These goals include improvements in education, housing, nutrition, water quality, and sanitation. The scope for international action on antibiotic resistance includes the amelioration of the conditions that potentiate the need for antibiotics and the spread of resistant forms of agents of infection. Improving living conditions (including housing), nutrition, education (for example with respect to risk factors for disease), and other determinants of human dignity such as female empowerment have been shown to reduce the risk of stunting, but these are also important factors in the control of infectious disease transmission and potentially antibiotic resistance. Achieving UN Development Goals (assuming that fairly and honestly set – see Hickel 2017) for 2030 would do much to mitigate the risk factors for both stunting and the transmission of agents of infection in both antibiotic sensitive and resistant forms.

Conclusions

Nussbaum's capability theory (Nussbaum 2006) provides a rich and relevant evaluative space for framing antibiotic resistance. Securing child development and adult capabilities requires that we address inequalities in access, regulate 'appropriate prescribing', and clarify responsibilities for addressing inequalities in risk factors for the dissemination and transmission of antibiotic resistance. Historical and current patterns of antibiotic use impose a burden of responsibility on developed countries to ensure that their own use is appropriate, and raise questions with respect to the responsibilities of developed countries to address risk factors for antibiotic resistant infection in developing countries. Antibiotics and antibiotic resistant bacteria pollute the environment (particularly when sanitation standards are poor) – compounding the inequality and disadvantage of those without equivalent access to effective antibiotics. Inequality undermines the cooperative activity that is control of infectious diseases and compounds the threat to the securing of child development and adult capabilities that comes from antibiotic resistance.

Note 1
There is some empirical evidence that European countries with more income inequality have higher levels of antibiotic resistance than those with less inequality (Kirby and Herbert 2013). Lack of access to high quality data makes this relationship difficult to study more generally.

Note 2
For Scanlon, reasons are facts (Scanlon 2014, p. 30, note 20), natural (e.g., that you will enjoy some activity) or normative (e.g., a law's being unjust or your having reason to go on living; Scanlon 2014, p. 32). These facts are an essential part of a relation to an agent: consideration (or fact) p is a reason for x to do a in circumstances c. 'Is a reason for' is a four-place relation, R(p, x, c, a) (pp. 31, 37). For Scanlon there are cases where the relative strength of reasons is derived from the

relative amounts of something (such as capabilities), even so he considers it to be a mistake to consider that there must inevitably be a quantitative property which determines the relative strength of reasons (p. 110). 'The strength of a reason is an essentially comparative notion, understood only in relation to other particular reasons' (p. 111). When we judge that certain considerations provide conclusive reasons for (or against) certain actions in certain circumstances, justification comes our understanding of a relationship with other rational beings that we have reason to want, specifically, the relationship of seeing them as beings to whom justification is owed (p. 115). Scanlon acknowledges that 'when we are assessing the justifiability of moral principles we must have reason to appeal to things that individuals have reason to want, and that many of these are things that contribute to well-being intuitively understood.' However, 'we cannot delimit the range of considerations that figure in justification by defining the boundaries of well-being' (Scanlon 1998, p. 140; see Putnam 2008).

Note 3

Scanlon emphasises the importance of probabilities in determining the degree of effort that we make to control risks. 'The probability that a form of conduct will cause harm can be relevant not as a factor diminishing the 'complaint' of the affected parties (discounting the harm by the likelihood of their suffering it) but rather as an indicator of the care that the agent has to take to avoid causing harm'. Scanlon states that '..the cost of avoiding all behaviour that involves risk of harm would be unacceptable. Our idea of 'reasonable precautions' defines the level of care that we think can be demanded: a principle that demanded more than this would be too confining, and could reasonably be rejected on that ground' (Scanlon 1998, p. 209 & pp. 235–6; see Kumar 2016). Scanlon's emphasis on reasons allows the inclusion of morally salient considerations such as responsibility and fairness (Scanlon 1998, p. 243). 'Responsibility of an agent for wrongful conduct, responsibility for creating a situation that gives reason to break a promise, responsibility for engaging in risky conduct that leads to harm and responsibility for misfortune that puts one in need of aid' (Scanlon 1998, p. 244) are all morally salient considerations. The question that arises is 'who has responsibility for 'reasonable precautions' when it comes to antibiotic resistance in developing countries', and what is reasonable?

Acknowledgement I'd like to thank Dr. Andrew Prendergast for raising the issue of growth stunting and the interaction with infectious disease.

References

Ahammad, Z.S., T.R. Sreekrishnan, C.L. Hands, C.W. Knapp, and D.W. Graham. 2014. Increased waterborne blaNDM-1 resistance gene abundances associated with seasonal human pilgrimages to the upper Ganges river. *Environmental Science & Technology* 48 (5): 3014–3020. https://doi.org/10.1021/es405348h.

Ashcroft, R.E. 2005. Making sense of dignity. *Journal of Medical Ethics* 31: 679–682.

Berendonk, T.U., C.M. Manaia, C. Merlin, D. Fatta-Kassinos, E. Cytryn, F. Walsh, H. Bürgmann, H. Sørum, M. Norström, M.N. Pons, N. Kreuzinger, P. Huovinen, S. Stefani, T. Schwartz, V. Kisand, F. Baquero, and J.L. Martinez. 2015. Tackling antibiotic resistance: The environmental framework. *Nature Reviews. Microbiology* 13 (5): 310–317. https://doi.org/10.1038/nrmicro3439.

Berrazeg, M., S.M. Diene, L. Medjahed, P. Parola, M. Drissi, D. Raoult, and J.M. Rolain. 2014. New Delhi metallo-beta-lactamase around the world: An eReview using Google Maps. *Eurosurveillance* 19 (20): pii=20809.

Biggeri, M., and S. Mehrotra. 2011. Child poverty as capability deprivation: How to choose domains of child well-being and poverty. In *Children and the capability approach*, ed. M. Biggeri, J. Ballet, and F. Comim. Basingstoke: Palgrave Macmillan.

Biggeri, M., J. Ballet, and F. Comim, eds. 2011. *Children and the capability approach*. Basingstoke: Palgrave Macmillan.

Black, R.E., C. Levin, N. Walker, D. Chou, M. Temmerman, and for the DCP3 RMNCH Authors Group. 2016. Reproductive, maternal, newborn, and child health: Key messages from disease control priorities 3rd edition. *Lancet* 388: 2811–2824.

Byrnes, J.P., D.C. Miller, and W.D. Schafer. 1999. Gender differences in risk taking: A meta-analysis. *Psychological Bulletin* 125: 367–383.

Casanovas, M.C., C. Lutter, N. Mangasaryan, R. Mwadime, N. Hajeebhoy, A.M. Aguilar, et al. 2013. Multisectoral interventions for healthy growth. *Maternal & Child Nutrition* 9 (Suppl.2): 46–57.

Centre for Science and Environment Report. (2014). www.cseindia.org/node/5487

Chi, P., and X. Li. 2014. Impact of parental HIV/AIDS on children's psychological well-being: A systematic review of global literature. *AIDS and Behavior* 17 (7): 2554–2574.

Chilton, M. 2006. Developing a measure of dignity for stress-related health outcomes. *Health and Human Rights* 9 (2): 208–233.

Comstock, G. 2000. Epidemiology of tuberculosis. In *Tuberculosis: A comprehensive international approach*, ed. L.B. Reichman and E.S. Hershfield, 129–156. New York: Marcel Dekker.

Ethier, K.A., T.S. Kershaw, J.B. Lewis, S. Milan, L.M. Niccolai, and J.R. Ickovics. 2006. Self-esteem, emotional distress and sexual behavior among adolescent females: Inter-relationships and temporal effects. *The Journal of Adolescent Health* 38 (3): 268–274.

Fitzpatrick, T. 2008. From contracts to capabilities and back again. *Research Publications* 14: 83–100.

Gough, E.K., E.E.M. Moodie, A.J. Prendergast, S.M.A. Johnson, J.H. Humphrey, R.J. Stoltzfus, A.S. Walker, I. Trehan, D.M. Gibb, R. Goto, S. Tahan, M.B. de Morais, and A.R. Manges. 2014. The impact of antibiotics on growth in children in low and middle income countries: Systematic review and meta-analysis of randomised controlled trials. *BMJ* 348: g2267.

Hair, N.L., J.L. Hanson, B.L. Wolfe, and S.D. Pollak. 2015. Association of child poverty, brain development, and academic achievement. *JAMA Pediatrics* 169 (9): 822–829. https://doi.org/10.1001/jamapediatrics.

Hickel, J. 2017. *The divide: A brief guide to global inequality and its solutions*. London: William Heinemann Ltd.

Horton, S., and R. Steckel. 2013. Global economic losses attributable to malnutrition 1900–2000 and projections to 2050. In *The economics of human challenges*, ed. B. Lomborg. Cambridge: Cambridge University Press.

Institute of Medicine. 2010. *Antibiotic resistance. Implications for global health and novel intervention strategies workshop summary*, Institute of Medicine (US) Forum on Microbial Threats. Washington, DC: National Academies Press (US).

International Leprosy Association – history of leprosy: leprosy and the family. Available at http://leprosyhistory.org/impact/leprosy-and-the-family. Accessed July 2017.

Kirby, A., and A. Herbert. 2013. Correlations between income inequality and antimicrobial resistance. *PLoS One* 8 (8): e73115. https://doi.org/10.1371/journal.pone.0073115.

Kumar, R. 2016. Risking and wronging. *Philosophy and Public Affairs* 43 (1): 27–51.

Kumarasamy, K.K., M.A. Toleman, T.R. Walsh, J. Bagaria, F. Butt, R. Balakrishnana, U. Chaudhary, et al. 2010. Emergence of a new antibiotic resistance mechanism in India, Pakistan, and the UK: A molecular, biological, and epidemiological study. *The Lancet Infectious Diseases* 10 (9): 597–602.

Laxminarayan, R., and R.R. Chaudhury. 2016. Antibiotic resistance in India: Drivers and opportunities for action. *PLoS Medicine* 13 (3): e1001974.

Laxminarayan, R., P. Matsoso, S. Pant, C. Brower, J.-A. Rottingen, K. Klugman, and S. Davies. 2016. Access to effective antimicrobials: A worldwide challenge. *Lancet* 387: 168–175.

Lübbert, C., C. Baars, A. Dayakar, N. Lippmann, A.C. Rodloff, M. Kinzig, and F. Sörgel. 2017. Environmental pollution with antimicrobial agents from bulk drug manufacturing industries in Hyderabad, South India is associated with dissemination of extended-spectrum beta-lactamase and carbapenemase-producing pathogens. *Infection* 45: 479–491. https://doi.org/10.1007/s15010-017-1007-2.

Mann, J. 1998. Dignity and health: The UDHR's revolutionary first article. *Health and Human Rights* 3 (2): 30–38.

Marmot, M. 2003. Self-esteem and health. *British Medical Journal* 327: 574–575.

———. 2005. Social determinants of health inequalities. *Lancet* 365: 1099–1104.

Millar, M. 2012. Constraining the use of antibiotics: Applying Scanlon's contractualism. *Journal of Medical Ethics* 38 (8): 465–469.

Noble, K.G., S.M. Houston, N.H. Brito, H. Bartsch, E. Kan, J.M. Kuperman, N. Akshoomoff, D.G. Amaral, C.S. Bloss, O. Libiger, N.J. Schork, S.S. Murray, B.J. Casey, L. Chang, T.M. Ernst, J.A. Frazier, J.R. Gruen, D.N. Kennedy, P. Van Zijl, S. Mostofsky, W.E. Kaufmann, T. Kenet, A.M. Dale, T.L. Jernigan, and E.R. Sowell. 2015. Family income, parental education and brain structure in children and adolescents. *Nature Neuroscience* 18 (5): 773–778. https://doi.org/10.1038/nn.3983.

Nussbaum, M. 2006. *Frontiers of justice*. Cambridge, MA: Harvard University Press.

———. 2011. *Creating capabilities: The human development approach*. Cambridge, MA: Harvard University Press.

Nussbaum, M., and R. Dixon. 2012. *Children's rights and a capabilities approach: The question of special priority*, University of Chicago Public Law and Legal Theory Working Paper, No.384. Chicago: University of Chicago Law School.

O'Neill, M. 2013. Constructing a contractualist egalitarianism: Equality after Scanlon. *Journal of Moral Philosophy* 10: 429–461.

Pandey G. 2010. India rejects UK scientists' 'superbug' claim. *BBC News*.

Peleg, N. 2013. Reconceptualising the child's right to development: Children and the capability approach. *International Journal of Children's Rights* 21: 523–542.

Picket, K., and R. Wilkinson. 2010. *The spirit level: Why equality is better for everyone*. New York: Bloomsbury Press.

Ploug, T., S. Holm, and M. Gjerriset. 2015. The stigmatization dilemma in public health policy-the case of MRSA in Denmark. *BMC Public Health* 15: 640. https://doi.org/10.1186/s12889-015-2004-y.

Putnam, H. 2008. Capabilities and two ethical theories. *Journal of Human Development* 9: 377–388.

Rump, B., M. De Boer, R. Reis, M. Wassenberg, and J. van Steenbergen. 2017. Signs of stigma and poor mental health among carriers of MRSA. *The Journal of Hospital Infection* 95 (3): 268–274.

Scanlon, T.M. 1998. *What we owe to each other*. Cambridge, MA: Harvard University Press.

———. 2003. The diversity of objections to inequality. In *The difficulty of tolerance*. Cambridge: Cambridge University Press.

———. 2004. Lecture. When does equality matter? Unpublished paper. Available at http://www.politicalscience.stanford.edu/politicaltheoryworkshop/0607papers/scanlonpaper.pdf. Accessed May 2017.

———. 2006. Justice, responsibility, and the demands of equality. In *The egalitarian conscience: Essays in honour of G. A. Cohen*, ed. Christine Sypnowich, 70–87. Oxford: Oxford University Press.

———. 2013. Reply to Martin O'Neill. *Journal of Moral Philosophy* 10: 462–464.
———. 2014. *Being realistic about reasons*. Oxford: Oxford University Press.
———. (not dated). Lecture. Why does inequality matter? Available at https://www.law.berkeley.edu/wp-content/uploads/2016/01/Why-Does-Inequality-Matter-Chapters-8-9.pdf. Accessed May 2017.
Sedyaningsih, E.R., S. Isfandari, T. Soendoro, and S.F. Supari. 2008. Towards mutual trust, transparency and equity in virus sharing mechanism: The avian influenza case of Indonesia. *Annals of the Academy of Medicine, Singapore* 37: 482–488.
Sen, A. 1999. *Development as freedom*. New York: Random House.
Shelter. 2006. Chance of a lifetime: The impact of bad housing on children's lives. https://england.shelter.org.uk/__data/assets/pdf_file/.../Chance_of_a_Lifetime.pdf. Accessed June 2017.
Shultziner, D., and I. Rabinovici. 2011. Human dignity, self-worth, and humiliation: A comparative legal–psychological approach. *Psychology, Public Policy, and Law* 18 (1): 105. Available at: http://works.bepress.com/doron_shultziner/20/. Accessed May 2017.
Sinhal K. 2011. Lancet says sorry for 'Delhi bug'. *The Times of India*.
———. 2015. British medical journal *Lancet* to take Modi to task for ignoring health sector. *The Times of India*.
Sontag, S. 1989. *AIDS and its metaphors*. New York: Farrar, Straus and Giroux.
Stewart, C.P., L. Ianotti, K.G. Dewey, K.F. Michaelsen, and A.W. Onyango. 2013. Contextualising complementary feeding in a broader framework for stunting prevention. *Maternal & Child Nutrition* 9: 27–45.
Sugden J. 2013. India has lost superbug war. *Wall Street Journal*.
Tversky, A., and D. Kahneman. 1981. The framing of decisions and the psychology of choice. *Science* 211 (4481): 453–458.
United Nations. 1996. *International covenant on economic, social and cultural rights*. Geneva: United Nations.
———. 2014. *The road to dignity by 2030*. Geneva: United Nations.
———. 2015. Framework Convention on Climate Change UNFCCC, Decision 1/CP.21, Adoption of the Paris Agreement, UN Doc. FCCC/CP/2015/10/Add.1.
Upshur, R., J. Singh, and N. Ford. 2009. Apocalypse or redemption: Responding to extensively drug-resistant tuberculosis. *Bulletin of the World Health Organization* 87: 481–483. https://doi.org/10.2471/BLT.08.051698.
Van Boeckel, T.P., S. Gandra, A. Ashok, Q. Caudron, B.T. Grenfell, S.A. Levin, and R. Laxminarayan. 2014. Global antibiotic consumption 2000–2010; an analysis of national pharmaceutical sales data. *Lancet Infectious Diseases* 14: 742–750.
Van Boeckel, T.P., C. Brower, M. Gilbert, B.T. Grenfella, S.A. Levina, T.P. Robinsoni, A. Teillanta, and R. Laxminarayan. 2015. Global trends in antimicrobial use in food animals. *PNAS* 112 (18): 5649–5654.
Venkatapuran, S. 2011. *Health justice*. Cambridge: Polity Press.
———. 2013. Health, vital goals, and central human capabilities. *Bioethics* 27 (5): 271–279.
Wolff, J., and A. De-Shalit. 2007. *Disadvantage*. Oxford: Oxford University Press.
World Health Assembly. 2011. *Report of the open-ended working group of member states on pandemic influenza preparedness: Sharing of influenza viruses and access to vaccines and other benefits*, 64th World Health Assembly A64/8. Geneva: World Health Association.
World Health Organisation. 2005. *Strengthening health security by implementing the international health regulations*. Geneva: World Health Organisation.
———. 2013. Pneumonia still responsible for one fifth of child deaths. http://www.who.int/mediacentre/news/releases/2013/world-pneumonia-day-20131112/en/. Accessed May 2017.
———. 2014. *Antimicrobial resistance: global report on surveillance*. Geneva: World Health Organisation.
———. 2015. *Global action plan on antimicrobial resistance*. Geneva: World Health Organisation.
World health Organisation. Factsheet 392. Available at http://www.who.int/mediacentre/factsheets/fs392/en/. Accessed May 2017.

4

The Economics of Resistance Through an Ethical Lens

Richard D. Smith and Joanna Coast

Abstract Economics is concerned with the analysis of choice and the efficient use of resources. Markets for antibiotics are heavily affected by their 'public good' nature and the externality that results from their consumption in terms of resistance. The non-excludability and non-rivalry associated with knowledge production in antibiotic development also has implications for the supply of antibiotics. On the demand side there are ethical issues associated with free-riding by consumers, free-riding across nations and free-riding across time. On the supply side, the lack of a pipeline for new antibiotics for the future causes both ethical and economic issues – and from both perspectives, efforts should perhaps focus more on alternatives to antibiotics and adjustments to heath care systems to reduce reliance on antibiotics. Indeed, unlike many areas of health care, where economics and ethical perspectives may differ, antimicrobial resistance is a case where the two perspectives align in terms of ensuring efficient and sustainable development and use of this precious resources. All strategies for dealing with resistance should share the same goals of achieving an optimal balance in the use of antimicrobial agents and explicit consideration of the distributional implications.

Keywords Economics · Externalities · Public-goods · Free-riding · Discounting

Introduction

Antimicrobial resistance has finally come to the fore on national and international agendas, and is now recognised as a critical threat to public health, modern health systems, and economies (Smith 2015) [Ref: Chap. 1]. Although the broad potential

R. D. Smith (✉)
College of Medicine and Health, University of Exeter, Exeter, UK
e-mail: rich.smith@exeter.ac.uk

J. Coast
Population Health Sciences, Bristol Medical School, University of Bristol, Bristol, UK

impacts of resistance are clear – that less effective treatments means greater morbidity and mortality, more expensive treatments or hospital care, and more time off work – robust evidence on the extent of likely impacts of resistance on population health, health care and economies remains relatively limited and often contentious (Coast et al. 1996, 2002; O'Neill 2014; Smith and Coast 2013; Wilton et al. 2002). Like climate change, this lack of clarity stems from inherent uncertainty; in the case of resistance, relating to uncertainties around the growth path of resistance over time, the functional form of the relationship between resistance and antibiotic use, and estimates of the direct morbidity and mortality impacts attributable to resistance rather than underlying infection or other causes (Cormican and Vellinga 2012; Courvalin 2008).

However, apart from such uncertainties, a significant issue is the nature of the decision- making around the production and consumption of antibiotics. Although an intrinsically biological phenomenon, the conditions promoting, or mitigating against, the development and spread of antimicrobial resistance are shaped by choices that are made by farmers and vets, doctors and patients, industry and governments, amongst others, concerning what antibiotics to produce, purchase and use (Smith 2015). Economics, at its foundation, is concerned with analysing and evaluating such choices: what and why certain choices are made over others; the conditions under which such choices are made, and how different conditions affect those choices; and, crucially, whether these choices are the 'best' ones (that is, whether they are 'efficient' in the sense that no greater benefit could be gained from another choice that was available).

These choices are determined through some sort of 'market', broadly defined as a place (physical or virtual) where goods are traded. In this case, for example, a market is where patients and doctors will determine whether an antibiotic will be prescribed, or where a vet and a farmer agree on a course of action for sick animals. Regardless of whether money changes hands, this is the point where an antibiotic supplier will engage with the consumer. Markets also underpin whether, what and how much a producer may invest in production of antibiotics, and the price that the payer (the consumer or their agent, often governments or insurers in the case of healthcare) will pay.

However, markets for antibiotics are heavily affected by two forces which are important when considering the development of antimicrobial resistance and strategies to reduce resistance. First, there are significant 'public good' attributes to antibiotics that affect use and distribution. This means that markets, left alone, will 'fail'; that is, they will not result in a socially optimal level of either production or consumption of antibiotics (Smith and Coast 2003). Second, there are 'externality' effects – effects not included in the decision to consume – that are important, and again means that, left alone, the market will 'fail' and not result in a social optimum of antibiotic consumption (Coast et al. 1998).

Together, these two forces drive the under- and/or over-use of antibiotics compared to what is optimal from a societal perspective. This creates major issues for economic efficiency, as different choices would improve overall societal welfare, but also for ethics, in the sense that there will be equity impacts that create problems of distributive (in)justice in access to antibiotics and in the impact of antimicrobial resistance (Coast and Smith 2015).

This chapter describes the core *economic* features of antimicrobial resistance – the public good and externality forces – through an ethics 'lens', focussing especially on the resultant economic and ethical problems of free-riding in both production and consumption. The chapter begins with outlining the core economic perspective on antimicrobial resistance – the market, public goods and externalities – in more detail. From this basis, the chapter then turns to consider the specific issues related to the demand side and then the supply side, focussing on the ethics of the economics, and reflecting on possible strategies to address resistance. In particular, these sections consider the development of appropriate incentives by governments to address free-riding within countries and the development of appropriate incentives by international agencies to address free-riding across countries. Such incentive mechanisms are evaluated both in terms of their value in addressing the economic market- failure and their ethical implications. The chapter concludes with a brief reflection on antimicrobial resistance as a specific case where economic and ethical concerns converge.

Antimicrobial Resistance and 'The Market'

At its most fundamental, the market for antibiotics seeks to equate demand for them by patients (and farmers or those with pets, although in this chapter we will focus on use in humans only) with supply by providers (doctors, pharmacists or over-the-counter stores for example). Patients demand antibiotics because of the impact they (are believed to have) on a health issue, such as a sore throat or urinary-tract infection. There are well-known problems in the market for healthcare goods and services, including the lack of information held by the patient upon which to decide on whether, or how much, healthcare to demand, the resultant need of the patient to rely on an (in economic terminology) 'agent' (usually a medical professional) to help the patient decide on what to consume, and, often, the separation of the patient from payment through the role of a third-party funder – typically government or insurer (Guiness and Wiseman 2011). Markets in healthcare are, therefore, far from perfect, and thus often subject to government intervention in their provision and/or financing. These problems are also, at least partly, responsible for ethical concerns for distributive justice, as they can leave many individuals with no, or inadequate, access to healthcare. Over time, this has led to increased calls for initiatives to ensure 'universal health coverage'; it is now a major thrust of the World Health Organization and World Bank to deal with general market failures in healthcare and to increase access (World Health Organization 2015), whilst the specific market failures around antimicrobial resistance are dealt with through other agendas, such as the Sustainable Development Goals (Hanefeld et al. 2017).

Externalities

Beyond general issues of failure in healthcare markets, there are two specific features of the market for antibiotics that are significant in considering the generation of antimicrobial resistance, and in establishing policies to contain it (Coast et al. 1998). First, there are externality effects from the consumption of antibiotics. An externality is an effect that is outside of the immediate producer or consumer, and thus does not influence decision-making in the choice about whether to produce or consume that antibiotic. So, for the patient, the direct (expected) benefit of the antibiotic in treating an infection informs his or her decision, as do possible side-effects from taking it, along with any monetary cost associated with its purchase. However, a 'positive externality' that is not generally expected to be taken into account by this patient is the benefit to those individuals who would, in the absence of antibiotics, have been infected by them – that is, there is an external benefit associated with reduced transmission of pathogens. The existence of this positive externality means that, the market will under-provide antibiotics; it might be a good reason for a subsidy or other policy to reduce the private cost to individuals. There is also an ethical issue involved here. There is a responsibility for each individual to consider the impact of their choice about receiving treatment on the wider community – that part of their decision to take treatment should, morally, include consideration of the impact of (reduced) infection on the wider population.

More critically for the discussion here is that there is also a major 'negative' externality from consumption of antibiotics – antimicrobial resistance. It is important to note that this externality is not associated with the production of antibiotics but with their consumption. The effects of antibiotic use, in terms of the sustained effectiveness of that antibiotic for others, or for the same individual in the future, do not influence the costs that must be paid by the patient, nor the benefits to them of taking the antibiotic now. They are therefore unlikely to be considered in the decision to purchase and consume that antibiotic (by either the patient or the health professional acting as their agent). From a societal perspective there is thus an over-consumption of antibiotics. Again, there are distributive issues here around the use of a limited resource knowing that it will generate possible greater ill-health in the future and/or for others.

On balance, the optimal consumption of antibiotics from a societal perspective is a balance of the costs and benefits that accrue directly to the individual concerned, plus these external benefits and costs to society (Coast et al. 1998). In recent years, consensus has been that on balance there is over-consumption – that the private costs and benefits and the positive externality are being severely compromised by not accounting for the negative externality of resistance. Focus has therefore been to see how these external costs of resistance can be internalised in to the decision to consume (in addition to how to increase the supply of effective antibiotics). We look at these strategies – affecting the demand and supply sides respectively – later in this chapter.

Public Goods

Second, there are 'public good' aspects associated with antibiotics [Ref: Chap. 8]. Most goods are what we term as 'private' in nature: their consumption can be withheld until a payment is made in exchange, and once consumed they cannot be consumed again (Woodward and Smith 2003). For example, the consumption of a cake can be withheld from the consumer until the consumer pays the baker a price, and once the consumer has eaten that cake it cannot be eaten again. A private good is therefore considered 'excludable' and 'rival in consumption'. At the other end of the spectrum lie public goods, which are defined as having the opposite characteristics. That is, the benefits, once the good is provided, cannot be restricted and are therefore available to all (i.e. non-excludable), and consumption by one individual does not limit consumption of that same good by others (i.e. non-rival in consumption). A classic example is the service provided by a lighthouse: the warning it provides is available to all who would benefit from it, and one ship's use of it does not limit the ability of other ships to use it. Virtually all public goods are such services or other intangibles, with few, if any, 'commodities' (in the narrow sense of physical objects) meeting these criteria (the exception to this being physical infrastructure, such as sewage systems, which once completed are largely non-rival in consumption, and difficult to exclude people from using).

However, both excludability and rivalry are relative, not absolute, concepts, and there is a scale of both rivalry and excludability. For example, access to public goods in particular may be specific to geography (e.g. conventional television broadcasts, while they broadly satisfy the criteria for a public good, reach only an area defined by the location of transmitters, the strength of signals and topographical constraints) or can be artificially made excludable (such as by using encryption services for satellite broadcasts). These create 'club goods', which are non-rival and are non-excludable to those who can access the 'club', but excludable to those outside of the club. Thus, some people could be (and often are) excluded from the benefits of most theoretically defined public goods through geographic, monetary or administrative prohibition. Similarly, rivalry in consumption may be relative to capacity, particularly in the case of physical infrastructure. For example, if a sewage system has spare capacity its use is non-rival, but as the capacity constraint is approached, its use becomes rivalrous; that person whose use of it causes capacity to be reached has effectively prevented the next person wishing to use it from doing so. Perhaps more usual is that the consumption of a particular good may not prevent others from using it, but simply reduces the benefits available. For example, one person's use of a road does not usually prevent use by others, but the use of the road becomes less beneficial as more and more people use it and the road consequently becomes more congested. This is sometimes termed the 'tragedy of the commons' (Hardin 1968), Chap. 8.

Of key importance, is that 'markets' under-supply public goods. First, non-excludability means that a price cannot be enforced, leading to 'free-riding' (one person can benefit from the actions of another person without reciprocation) and thus there is no incentive for anyone to produce or purchase the good. Second, non-rivalry means that the socially optimal level of consumption is far greater than the level that occurs at the 'market price' (Smith and Coast 2003).

To be clear, antibiotics are not themselves public goods – they can be made excludable, and they are rival in the sense that if I use one dose no one else can use that exact same dose.

However, the knowledge they embody in their development, and the resultant property of reduced infection (bearing in mind the externality properties above) means that they have significant public good attributes associated with them. Once developed, the knowledge required to produce the antibiotic can be made (virtually) freely available as dissemination of it is quick and cheap, and any one firm using it to produce the antibiotic does not prevent another from doing so. We will return to this aspect in the section concerning the supply of antibiotics in light of resistance. It also means that the benefits resulting from the consumption of the antibiotic, of reduced infection, cannot be made excludable – we all benefit from reduced transmission of pathogens – and is non-rival – my benefiting from this reduced risk of infection does not diminish you equally benefitting from it. And vice-versa – the reduced effectiveness of antibiotics due to resistance is also non-rival and non-excludable. It is this consumption side to which we now turn.

The Ethics and Economics of Demand

The characteristics of non-excludability and non-rivalry have important implications for the economics and ethics of the demand/consumption side of the market for antibiotics from a number of perspectives.

Free-Riding by Consumers

Consumers have an incentive to engage in free-riding, meaning that they have no incentive to reduce their own use of antibiotics, but rather to wait for others to do so, Chap. 21. This is perhaps also seen as morally acceptable as each individual consumption of each individual course of antibiotics will only add infinitesimally to the problem of resistance; an individual's personal consumption of antibiotics really is a 'drop in the ocean' relative to the total consumption of antimicrobials (Smith and Coast 2013). There are strong parallels here with climate change of course. Overall, the antimicrobial resistance problem is the accumulation of many millions of decisions by different decision makers for different patients in different health systems and facing different personal, financial and organizational incentives. Economic policies in general aim to induce consumers to internalize the costs of any negative externality, but because of the huge diffusion of the problem in relation to resistance, such policies may be very challenging if even possible at all.

For example, system interventions to address free-riding include taxation (akin to Pigovian taxes or pollution charges in the case of climate change), subsidy, permits or regulation (Coast et al. 1998; Laxminarayan et al. 2010; Smith and Coast 1998) although each of these would have their own distributional implications (Coast and Smith 2015), Chap. 8. Examples of clinical interventions that may address this issue may include better diagnostics (Kolmos and Little 1999; Oppong et al. 2013; Rice 2011) or educational campaigns providing better information (Goossens et al. 2006; Huttner et al. 2010), combined with a gatekeeping role from healthcare providers. Other possibilities include focussing more on assessing option or existence value (the idea that individuals have some personal utility from knowing that the option for them to consume antimicrobials in the future will be retained) (Coast et al. 2006). However, it is more likely that benefits may come from encouraging a greater moral responsibility to avoid resistance within society, such as has been undertaken with climate change and pollution, or as a parallel to stronger regulations, such as with banning smoking in public places, compulsory wearing of seatbelts in cars or drink-driving campaigns.

Free-Riding Across Nations

These issues of individual free-riding are also paralleled by free-riding across macro-settings. Actions taken by current patients have the potential to transmit resistance, through the pathogen this resistance is associated with, across international, cultural and ethnic boundaries. Antimicrobial resistance does not respect regional or national boundaries, with resistant organisms being able to travel from one setting to another just as easily as sensitive ones (Smith and Coast 2002). Globalization has increased the rate at which infectious diseases can travel, and resistances identified in one area are rapidly found in other countries and on other continents. Such spread will be dependent on many epidemiological factors, including for example, socio-demographic factors, density of the population, natural disasters, hygiene levels and so on. Areas with greater poverty may be particularly susceptible to the rapid spread of infection and thus the deleterious effects of resistance.

Transmission of resistance may have particularly severe consequences for economies which already suffer greatly from infectious disease – countries where living conditions are poor and where there are high proportions of individuals with immune-compromise – but it will also have significant economic and health consequences at a global level (Smith and Coast 2002).

Indeed, transmission of resistance across national boundaries compromises measures that individual countries may put in place to try to combat resistance; importing resistance from elsewhere may negate national initiatives, rendering them effectively pointless. Conversely, countries may do little to address resistance within their own borders, relying on the activities of other countries to reduce levels of resistance that come in and out of the country; effectively, individual countries may 'free-ride' on the actions of the wider global community and the containment policies operated in other settings. The potential for resistance to spread across boundaries reduces the incentive for any single country to act against resistance – either because it will appear futile in the face of a global rise in resistance, or because the optimal approach is to await every other country to act first – which means that none will.

The total effort devoted to containing antimicrobial resistance is thus likely to be suboptimal because some nations will rely on the efforts of other nations. This dilemma facing the creation of collective action against antimicrobial resistance at the global level has been highlighted elsewhere (Årdal et al. 2016; Smith and Coast 2002), although it has recently been suggested that international law may provide a means of dealing with the problem of collective action in this context (Hoffman et al. 2015a; Walls and Ooms 2017), Chaps. 24 and 25.

Despite the importance of the global issue in this context, economic (and other) assessments tend to be conducted on a national basis as if systems are closed to the outside world. Opening this up would promote awareness that it is in national self-interest to look to address resistance in other countries, and thus contribute to global initiatives, as well as be open to moral arguments, such as those that drive considerable development funds each year from developed to less developed nations (Molzon et al. 2011).

Time Preference and Discounting: Free-Riding Across Time

The externality effect is also inter-generational, generating significant issues of inter- generational as well as regional equity. Actions taken by current patients will impact on the transmission and emergence of resistance for future generations, but with similar lack of incentive for either individual consumers or nation states to fully account for the impact of their decisions on others.

The relevant economic concept here is that of time-preference and discounting – that people place higher weight on benefits that occur now and costs that occur in the future, thus biasing decisions and choices against future generations (even including themselves in that future generation). The discount rate is the amount at which future years are 'discounted', where a rate of 0 would give equal weight to the current and any future year, and 100% would give total weight to the current year and count future years as worthless. Thus, a higher rate places more weight on the present. Empirical literature finds huge variance in expressed discount rates, but this is overwhelmingly based on personal perspectives (Asenso-Boadi et al. 2008). These, typically high, rates are not consistent with the normative arguments that are considered when intergenerational equity is discussed, and less weighting explicitly given to current generations (Olsen and Richardson 2013; Richardson and McKie 2007). The authors have also previously noted that discount rates with respect to antimicrobial resistance "should reflect collective value judgements and moral issues, rather than just the preference that individuals have for their own consumption over time" (Coast et al. 1996). This is important as high discount rates would result in an almost exclusive focus on the current population, and would probably also mean that the focus would be on interventions intended to reduce transmission of antimicrobial resistance, which has relatively short-term gains, rather than interventions intended to reduce emergence of new resistances, which may be further down the line (but where the total benefits in the absence of discounting may be much greater). This issue is examined in greater detail elsewhere (Coast et al. 2002).

The Importance of Context

On the consumption side, therefore, the focus of policy is on incentives and systems to influence demand through education of patients, restriction of availability through regulation, or greater guidance to providers (Dar et al. 2016). There are huge challenges in this respect, not only of construction, enforcement and evaluation of any single policy, but also across contexts. Policy in most developed countries is concerned with reducing the over-use of antibiotics – their use where there is little or no clinical indication, such as for the common cold, their use where there is marginal clinical benefit (e.g. many minor infections in otherwise healthy people, which may hasten their cure by a few days only) and even use where there may be greater morbidity but the disease is not fatal. In contrast in many low- and middle-income countries the challenges are to increase use, where appropriate, to reduce pools of infection, and to reduce practices of dose splitting, use of sub-standard, out-of-date or counterfeit medicines, and cross use of antibiotics for humans and animals (Review on antimicrobial resistance 2015a).

The Ethics and Economics of Supply

Externality and public good aspects are not only relevant to consumers, but also to the producers of antibiotics. The supply-chain of antibiotics is long – from original discovery, research and development, which may be in universities, through testing and eventual production by a pharmaceutical company, through wholesalers, health systems or private pharmacy and retailers (with prospects for counterfeit or sub-standard antibiotics being introduced along the way), Chap. 5 However, critical to this discussion is the core discovery, development and production of the antibiotics; especially that undertaken in the private sector.

It has been noted many times that there has been a distinctly dry pipeline for new antibiotics over recent decades, with no new class of antibiotic being discovered for many years and declining investment by the pharmaceutical industry in the area of anti-infectives (Cormican and Vellinga 2012). What underlies this is the current business model for the development of pharmaceuticals, which is based on a market response to 'free-riding' (Smith et al. 2009).

Free-Riding and Intellectual Property

Basic research and development of new drugs is hugely expensive, but the information that is produced from this research and development activity – such as the chemical formulation of a new antibiotic – is almost costless to disseminate, is very hard (especially in the internet age) to exclude other companies having access to, and is non-rival in the sense that me using this information to produce the drug does not prevent you also using the information to produce the drug. Thus, given the non-excludability of this information, it is socially optimal to encourage wide dissemination and use of it, which can be achieved at almost zero cost once produced. But, the inability to exclude means that a high-price cannot be charged for it to recoup the original investment in its production, and so other producers can 'free-ride' on the back of the one who first produced the information. Since the original producers cannot recoup their costs, let alone gain a profit, then there is no incentive for that information to be produced. Hence, left to this pure market system, there would be no medicines developed (Smith and Coast 2003).

The 'solution' to this situation has been to develop an artificial exclusion system to enable the original producer who discovers and develops the information to charge a higher price to compensate for the research and development costs incurred. This is the 'Intellectual Property Right' system, which in the case of pharmaceuticals is operationalised through a patent (Smith et al. 2009). This system confers a legal exclusion to be placed on others using material that is patented for a specified number of years – usually 20–30. During this time whoever filed the patent, such as the pharmaceutical company, has exclusive rights to use it and can therefore charge a sufficiently high price for the medicine it develops from it to allow it to recoup the costs invested, and to make a profit (Yamabhai and Smith 2015).

This 'solution', however, creates a critical problem for both efficiency and ethics. Due to the non-rival nature of the information – and the non-rival nature of the resultant reduction in infectious disease risk from taking the antibiotic that is based on the information – it is most socially efficient if it is widely disseminated and used. The patent system creates a restriction on that use, since only those who can afford to pay the price now charged can access it, which will be at a level lower than is socially optimal. Ethically, it also means that the information – and resultant antibiotics – are only available at a much higher price than the production cost, with the known consequence that there will be people who can benefit who are being denied that treatment (Mendelson et al. 2016). The 'patent wedge' between cost price and the price charged by the patent holder can typically by seen when the patent period expires and 'generic' versions of branded pharmaceuticals are made available, which are often hundreds of times cheaper (Smith et al. 2009). During the patent period there are clearly therefore poorer people, and countries, that are not able to afford to access these drugs and where ill-health is suffered as a result. For example, the most infamous case is that relating to anti-retroviral therapies for HIV/AIDS which were priced at over US$10,000 per person per year by those producing branded products, but could be produced by generic manufacturers for US$365 per patient per year (Keppler 2013). This is both inefficient and unethical (Laxminarayan et al. 2016). Inequality in access due to price – especially for those in low-income settings – has been the cause of considerable debate more widely with respect to medicines (Trouiller et al. 2002).

There is added complexity in the case of antibiotics, compared to other medicines, in part due to the nature of antibiotics, which are relatively inexpensive compared to other drugs that could be developed and are used for short periods of time (thus reducing the potential profit), and in part due to the development of resistance, as polices elsewhere seek to reduce and restrict use. This is especially the case in high-income countries, which is where the major markets for new antibiotics are based and where companies expect to be able to charge the higher-prices required to support research and development. The combination then of the high development cost, with reduced market volume, has discouraged investment in this area.

Alternative Systems

Over the years there have been growing calls for changes to the patent system as underpinning research and development in pharmaceutical in general, largely from those concerned about the bias towards health needs of high-income countries who are the major markets, resulting in concerns around 'neglected diseases' (Trouiller et al. 2002), Chap. 10. More recently, especially following the report from the Independent Review on Antimicrobial Resistance, chaired by Lord Jim O'Neill, there has been a renewed push for the development of new systems for incentivising investment in new antibiotics, where high-income countries too have considerable need that is not being met (Review on antimicrobial resistance 2015a).

One popular alternative is the de-linking of profitability from sales volumes (Brogan and Mossialos 2016; Review on antimicrobial resistance 2015b; Wise 2015). For example, pre- purchase agreements could be made by governments to guarantee the pharmaceutical company a minimum 'market' in terms of sales, but then the government can choose whether and how those drugs would be disseminated. This builds on other recent work, such as by Chatham House, a think-tank on international affairs, which has outlined alternative business models to similarly change the current financial models for encouraging and supporting research and development in new antibiotics (Kesselheim and Outterson 2010; Outterson 2014; Outterson et al. 2015). There is a lot of work and funding also now going in to research and development by governments themselves to directly develop new antibiotics. For example, The U.S. granted GlaxoSmithKline US$200 million for investment in new antibiotic research and development (GlaxoSmithKline 2013). There are also other initiatives. In the United States for instance there has been an extension to marketing exclusivity, accelerated review, and a relaxation of requirements for approval by the Food and Drug Administration (Hatch 2015). Although this leniency may have increased the development and launch of new antibiotics, there is worrying evidence that such 'fast tracking' may generate considerable adverse effects (Doshi 2015).

Critical, of course, is the basic fact that because resistance to an antibiotic begins as soon as it is developed, new agents can never be the sole solution—and are unlikely to be the most cost-effective or sustainable, Chap. 19. Thus, in addition to looking at encouragement of new drug discovery, another focus has been on initiatives to support the sustainable use of current antibiotics through the development of rapid diagnostic tests to support the more 'appropriate' use of antibiotics (Review on antimicrobial resistance 2015a). In the UK there have been specific funds made available to support diagnostics research and development through the UK Research Councils (Medical Research Council 2014), and the Longitude Prize, where £1 m is to be awarded to whoever first develops a specific rapid – and affordable – diagnostic tool (Nesta 2014). The critical issue here is the last one – affordability. Diagnostic tests face a challenge of affordability in relation to the option to simply take the – currently cheaper – antibiotic. The cost of the test relative to the cost of the antibiotic is critical – if the test costs more than, or even approximates, the antibiotic cost then it is likely to be rational for individuals to simply take the antibiotic and risk it not working – if it does work they save the cost of the test, if it does not work then they may need another drug but have still saved the cost of the test, whereas if they have the test and don't need an antibiotic they may have incurred a cost greater than that of simply taking the antibiotic, and if the test suggests they do need that antibiotic all they have done is add a cost of the test on to what they would have paid in any case. There are challenges especially for this in community settings, rather than hospitals, and in low- and middle-income countries.

Given that a critical feature of antimicrobial resistance is that it occurs naturally for all antibiotics, developing new drugs may win successive battles but not the war. It is possible that genomic developments may produce antibiotics where resistance is not seen, or new ways to tackle pathogens. However, in the absence of those, the most serious issue is not, perhaps, systems for encouraging development in new technologies, but rather how to design health systems that are less reliant on antibiotics. Modern healthcare especially, has been built on the basis that infections can be prevented or treated easily and cheaply. Healthcare has become increasingly technological and invasive, and antibiotics have become integrated in many aspects of care, from prevention of iatrogenic infection in surgery, to women delivering by caesarean section to those having cancer treatment (Smith 2015). From both economic and ethical perspectives efforts should perhaps focus more on alternatives to antibiotics and on adjustments to health systems and care pathways to reduce reliance upon antibiotics.

Discussion: The Convergence of Ethics and Economics

Far from the 'dismal science', or the often perceived amoral (if not immoral) nature of economics being in conflict with ethics, antimicrobial resistance is a case where the two perspectives are frequently aligned. Many of the economic imperatives for ensuring the efficient and sustainable development and use of antibiotics are in-line with major ethical principles to secure benefits that are equitably available and distributed. In this sense, from an economic and ethical perspective, we are seeking to:

- Develop alternative systems to support the discovery, development and production of new antibiotics that are effective for all major infectious diseases globally
- Ensure that these antibiotics are available to those populations that would benefit from them, wherever they are in the world
- Look for alternatives to reduce reliance on antibiotics – alternatives for the same treatment or prevention of infection, and alternatives to avoid infection and risk of infection and hence requirement for antibiotics or their substitutes

It is also important to note that, at least from an economics perspective, the 'eradication' of resistance is not necessarily a desirable goal. To eradicate resistance entirely – or even to maintain resistance at current levels – would require significant, if not total, reduction in the use of antibiotics, as the use of any antibiotic will lead to the development of some resistance.

Such a goal would imply allowing significant mortality and morbidity to be incurred – far in excess of that caused by the resistance itself. The aim must therefore be to use the available strategies to optimise the balance between the current use of effective antibiotics to treat infection, and thus reduce morbidity and mortality today, and minimising the emergence and spread of resistance to these antibiotics and the consequent increased future morbidity and mortality. This balance depends upon the relative costs and benefits of the positive and negative effects involved. It is determining this balance that is critical, and requires consideration from both an economics and an ethical perspective, as it encompasses significant inter-generational and inter-regional distributional aspects.

Given the diverse contexts of the developed and developing nations, it is likely that optimal strategies will vary considerably across these them, but all strategies should share the same goals of achieving an optimal balance in the use of antimicrobial agents (Hoffman et al. 2015b; Woolhouse and Farrar 2014) and explicit consideration of the distributional implications.

References

Årdal, C., K. Outterson, S.J. Hoffman, A. Ghafur, M. Sharland, N. Ranganathan, et al. 2016. International cooperation to improve access to and sustain effectiveness of antimicrobials. *The Lancet* 387 (10015): 296–307.

Asenso-Boadi, F., T.J. Peters, and J. Coast. 2008. Exploring differences in empirical time preference rates for health: An application of meta-regression. *Health Economics* 17: 235–248.

Brogan, D.M., and E. Mossialos. 2016. Systems, not pills: The options market for antibiotics seeks to rejuvenate the antibiotic pipeline. *Social Science & Medicine* 151: 167–172.

Coast, J., and R.D. Smith. 2015. Distributional considerations in economic responses to antimicrobial resistance. *Public Health Ethics* 8 (3): 225–237.

Coast, J., R.D. Smith, and M.R. Millar. 1996. Superbugs: Should antimicrobial resistance be included as a cost in economic evaluation? *Health Economics* 5: 217–226.

———. 1998. An economic perspective on policy to reduce antimicrobial resistance. *Social Science and Medicine* 46 (1): 29–38.

Coast, J., R.D. Smith, P. Wilton, A.M. Karcher, and M.R. Millar. 2002. Superbugs II: How should economic evaluation be conducted for interventions which aim to reduce antimicrobial resistance? *Health Economics* 11 (7).

Coast, J., R.D. Smith, and M.R. Millar. 2006. Disentangling value: Assessing the benefits of containing antimicrobial resistance. In *The economics of infectious disease*, ed. J.A. Roberts, 201–214. Oxford: Oxford University Press. (Reprinted from: In File).

Cormican, M., and A. Vellinga. 2012. Existing classes of antibiotics are probably the best we will ever have. *British Medical Journal* 344: e3369.

Courvalin, P. 2008. Predictable and unpredictable evolution of antibiotic resistance. *Journal of Internal Medicine* 264 (1): 4–16.

Dar, O.A., R. Hasan, J. Schlundt, S. Harbarth, G. Caleo, F.K. Dar, et al. 2016. Exploring the evidence base for national and regional policy interventions to combat resistance. *The Lancet* 387 (10015): 285–295.

Doshi, P. 2015. Speeding new antibiotics to market: A fake fix? *BMJ: British Medical Journal* 350: h1453.

GlaxoSmithKline. 2013. *GlaxoSmithKline awarded up to $200 million by U.S. Government to develop new antibiotics*. Middlesex: GlaxoSmithKline.

Goossens, H., D. Guillemot, M. Ferech, B. Schlemmer, M. Costers, M. Van Breda, L.J. Baker, et al. 2006. National campaigns to improve antibiotic use. *European Journal of Clincal Pharmacology* 62: 373–379.

Guiness, L., and V. Wiseman. 2011. *Introduction to health economics*. 2nd ed. Maidenhead: McGraw-Hill Education.

Hanefeld, J., M. Khan, G. Tomson, and R. Smith. 2017. Trade is central to achieving the sustainable development goals: A case study of antimicrobial resistance. *BMJ* 358: j3505.

Hardin, G. 1968. The tragedy of the commons. *Science* 162 (3859): 1243–1248.

Hatch, O. 2015. *Promise for antibiotics and therapeutics for health act or the PATH act*. In. www.congress.gov/bill/114th-congress/senate-bill/185?q=%7B%22search%22%3A%5B%22s.185%22%5D%7D.

Hoffman, S.J., K. Outterson, J.-A. Røttingen, O. Cars, C. Clift, Z. Rizvi, et al. 2015a. An international legal framework to address antimicrobial resistance. *Bulletin of the World Health Organization* 93 (2): 66–66.

Hoffman, S.J., J.-A. Røttingen, and J. Frenk. 2015b. Assessing proposals for new global health treaties: An analytic framework. *American Journal of Public Health* 105 (8): 1523–1530.

Huttner, B., H. Goossens, T. Verheij, and S. Harbarth. 2010. Characteristics and outcomes of public campaigns aimed at improving the use of antibiotics in outpatients in high- income countries. *Lancet Infectious Diseases* 10: 17–31.

Keppler, H. 2013. *The untold AIDS story: How access to antiretroviral drugs was obstruced in Africa*.

Kesselheim, A.S., and K. Outterson. 2010. Fighting antibiotic resistance: Marrying new financial incentives to meeting public health goals. *Health Affairs* 29 (9): 1689–1696.

Kolmos, H.J., and P. Little. 1999. Should general practitioners perform diagnostic tests on patients before prescribing antibiotics? *British Medical Journal* 318: 799–802.

Laxminarayan, R., I.W.H. Parry, D.L. Smith, and E.Y. Klein. 2010. Should new antimalarial drugs be subsidized? *Journal of Health Economics* 29: 445–456.

Laxminarayan, R., P. Matsoso, S. Pant, C. Brower, J.-A. Røttingen, K. Klugman, and S. Davies. 2016. Access to effective antimicrobials: A worldwide challenge. *The Lancet* 387 (10014): 168–175.

Medical Research Council. 2014. *Tackling AMR theme 2: Accelerating therapeutic and diagnostics development EOI.* In. www.mrc.ac.uk/funding/browse/tackling-amr-theme-2-accelerating-therapeutic-and-diagnostics-development-eoi.

Mendelson, M., J.-A. Røttingen, U. Gopinathan, D.H. Hamer, H. Wertheim, B. Basnyat, et al. 2016. Maximising access to achieve appropriate human antimicrobial use in low-income and middle-income countries. *The Lancet* 387 (10014): 188–198.

Molzon, J.A., A. Giaquinto, L. Lindstrom, T. Tominaga, M. Ward, P. Doerr, et al. 2011. The value and benefits of the international conference on harmonisation to drug regulatory authorities: Advancing harmonization for better public health. *Clinical Pharmacology & Therapeutics* 89 (4): 503–512.

Nesta. 2014. *The challenge: Reduce the use of antibiotics.* In. https://longitudeprize.org/challenge.

O'Neill, J. 2014. *Review on antimicrobial resistance. Antimicrobial resistance: Tackling a crisis for the health and wealth of nations.* London: HM Government; Wellcome Trust.

Olsen, J.A., and J. Richardson. 2013. Preferences for the normative basis of health care priority setting: Some evidence from two countries. *Health Economics* 22 (4): 480–485.

Oppong, R., M. Jit, R.D. Smith, C.C. Butler, H. Melbye, S. Molstad, and J. Coast. 2013. Cost-effectiveness of point-of-care C-reactive protein testing to inform antibiotic prescribing decisions. *British Journal of General Practice* 63 (612): e465–e471.

Outterson, K. 2014. *New business models for sustainable antibiotics.* London: Chatham House.

Outterson, K., J.H. Powers, G.W. Daniel, and M.B. McClellan. 2015. Repairing the broken market for antibiotic innovation. *Health Affairs* 34 (2): 277–285.

Review on antimicrobial resistance. 2015a. *Tackling a global health crisis: Initial steps.*

———. 2015b. *Securing new drugs for future generations: The pipeline of antibiotics.*

Rice, L.B. 2011. Rapid diagnostics and appropriate antibiotic use. *Clinical Infectious Diseases* 52 (Suppl 4): S357–S360.

Richardson, J., and J. McKie. 2007. Economics, political philosophy and ethics: The role of public preferences in health care decision–making. In *Principles of health care ethics*, 2nd ed., 569–576.

Smith, R. 2015. Antimicrobial resistance is a social problem requiring a social solution. *BMJ: British Medical Journal* 350: h1453.

Smith, R.D., and J. Coast. 1998. Controlling antimicrobial resistance: A proposed transferable permit market. *Health Policy* 43: 219–232.

———. 2002. Antimicrobial resistance: a global response. *Bulletin of the World Health Organization* 80: 126–133.

———. 2003. Antimicrobial drug resistance. In *Global public goods for health: A health economic and public health perspective*, ed. R.D. Smith, R. Beaglehole, D. Woodward, and N. Drager. Oxford: Oxford University Press.

Smith, R., and J. Coast. 2013. The true cost of antimicrobial resistance. *BMJ* 346 (f1493): 1–5.

Smith, R.D., C. Carlos, and O. Cecilia. 2009. Trade, TRIPS, and pharmaceuticals. *Lancet* 373 (9664): 684–691.

Trouiller, P., P. Olliaro, E. Torreele, J. Orbinski, R. Laing, and N. Ford. 2002. Drug development for neglected diseases: A deficient market and a public-health policy failure. *The Lancet* 359 (9324): 2188–2194.

Walls, H.L., and G. Ooms. 2017. Innovative use of the law to address complex global health problems: Comment on the legal strength of international health instruments-what it brings to global health governance? *International Journal of Health Policy Management* 6.

Wilton, P., R.D. Smith, J. Coast, and M.R. Millar. 2002. Strategies to contain the emergence of antimicrobial resistance: A systematic review of effectiveness and cost- effectiveness. *Journal of Health Services Research and Policy* 7: 111–117.

Wise, J. 2015. Report calls for $2 bn global fund to kickstart antibiotic development. *BMJ: British Medical Journal* 350: h2635.

Woodward, D., and R.D. Smith. 2003. Global public goods for health: Concepts and issues. In *Global public goods for health: A health economic and public health perspective*, ed. R.D. Smith, R. Beaglehole, D. Woodward, and N. Drager. Oxford: Oxford University Press.

Woolhouse, M., and J. Farrar. 2014. Policy: An intergovernmental panel on antimicrobial resistance. *Nature* 509 (7502): 555–557.

World Health Organization. 2015. *Tracking universal health coverage: First global monitoring report*. Geneva: World Health Organization.

Yamabhai, I., and R.D. Smith. 2015. To what extent are pharmaceutical prices determined by patents? A case study of oncology medicines in Thailand. *Journal of Intellectual Property Rights* 20: 89–95.

5

Global Health Governance and Antimicrobial Resistance

Belinda Bennett and Jon Iredell

Abstract This chapter analyses the challenges and the adequacy of existing frameworks to provide a strong foundation to support global responses to antimicrobial resistance. Calls for global responses are indicative of a growing global commitment to seeking practical means of tackling the growing problem of antimicrobial resistance. While antimicrobial resistance is often conceptualised as an emergency, the application of the International Health Regulations, designed to govern responses to public health emergencies of international concern, remains unclear. Furthermore, there may be challenges for countries in developing and resourcing national approaches to address antimicrobial resistance. Clarity and agreement around definitions of key concepts related to antimicrobial resistance will also be essential to antibiotic stewardship and development of policy in this area. Finally, improvements to health systems as a result of the Sustainable Development Goals may help to support improvements in public health and may play a role in global strategies to address antimicrobial resistance.

Keywords Antimicrobial resistance · International Health Regulations · Sustainable Development Goals

Introduction

Antimicrobial resistance (AMR) has been described as 'a global health crisis,' (Review on Antimicrobial Resistance 2015) 'a slowly emerging disaster' (Viens and Littman 2015), and 'a complex global public health challenge' (World Health

---

B. Bennett (✉)
School of Law, Queensland University of Technology, Brisbane, Queensland, Australia
e-mail: belinda.bennett@qut.edu.au

J. Iredell
Department of Infectious Diseases, Westmead Hospital and University of Sydney, Sydney, NSW, Australia

Organization 2014: xix). With AMR raising the possibility that we could soon be living in a 'post-antibiotic era' (World Health Organization 2014: ix) and with recognition that AMR 'threatens the sustainability of the public health response to many communicable diseases, including tuberculosis, malaria and HIV/AIDS' (World Health Assembly 2014), there is increased international dialogue around the need to find practical global solutions for the looming crisis (Laxminarayan et al. 2013). Others have argued for the need for AMR strategies to address equitable *access* to medicines; *conservation* through stewardship and appropriate use of antimicrobials; and *innovation* to ensure the development of the new antimicrobials, as well as the importance of a binding legal framework addressing these issues (Hoffman, Outterson, Røttingen et al. 2015; Hoffman, Røttingen and Frenk 2015). Proposals have included a new international treaty (Hoffman, Outterson, Røttingen et al. 2015; Anomaly 2010), the establishment of an intergovernmental panel (Woolhouse and Farrar 2014), a range of policy options to support action on AMR (Hoffman, Caleo, Daulaire et al. 2015), and the use of the International Health Regulations as an existing framework for managing global health risks (Wernli et al. 2011). Such is the complexity of the challenge posed by AMR that national and regional approaches alone are unlikely to be effective solutions (Littman et al. 2020). Yet the complex nature of AMR presents considerable challenges for global health governance, and with recent global health crises revealing shortcomings in global health governance, there are clearly significant challenges associated with utilising existing frameworks to address the growing problem of AMR. This chapter analyses these challenges and the adequacy of existing frameworks to provide a strong foundation to support global action on AMR.

The Rise of Drug Resistance

Severe infection long ago overtook heart attacks in terms of likelihood of hospital admission in developed countries (Seymour et al. 2012). The ability to manage it is essential for intensive care, major surgery and transplantation services that are increasingly routine. Up to 20 million people each year are treated with mechanical ventilation in intensive care (Adhikari et al. 2010). Infection complicates about half of ICU admissions and is an important cause of death in the critically ill (Vincent et al. 2009).

Antibiotics are a cornerstone of treatment of severe infection, with the risk of death increasing in the presence of antibiotic resistance (Review on Antimicrobial Resistance 2016a). In response to the steady rise in antibiotic resistance that began soon after the first introduction of antibiotics and has been quickly accelerating (Davies et al. 2013; Laxminarayan et al. 2013; Review on Antimicrobial Resistance 2016a: 10), experts call for international co-ordination of public policy solutions that include (i) better antibiotic controls in industry, agriculture and medicine (antimicrobial stewardship), and (ii) better surveillance and containment (infection control) (Howard et al. 2013; Laxminarayan et al. 2013; Piddock 2012; Spellberg et al. 2008).

A Global Approach to AMR?

With the recognition of the problems posed by growing AMR have come calls for a global approach to limiting the spread of AMR and its associated risks. In 2015 the World Health Assembly adopted a global action plan on antimicrobial resistance (World Health Organization 2015a; Ho and Lee 2020) and called on Member States to develop national actions plans on AMR and to 'mobilize human and financial resources through domestic, bilateral and multilateral channels in order to implement plans and strategies in line with the global action plan' (World Health Assembly 2015). The global action plan included five strategic objectives:

> (1) to improve awareness and understanding of antimicrobial resistance; (2) to strengthen knowledge through surveillance and research; (3) to reduce the incidence of infection; (4) to optimize the use of antimicrobial agents; and (5) to ensure sustainable investment in countering antimicrobial resistance (World Health Organization 2015a: 1)

The World Health Assembly resolution was followed in 2016 by a declaration by the high-level meeting of the United Nations General Assembly on antimicrobial resistance. The declaration of the high-level meeting included committing to work nationally, regionally and globally to address AMR, and to mobilize funding and resources to support the development and implementation of national plans (United Nations General Assembly 2016).

These calls for global action on antimicrobial resistance indicate a growing global commitment to seeking practical means of tackling the growing problem of antimicrobial resistance. As Wernli et al. have pointed out, this growing focus on AMR 'also indicates that AMR has transformed into a global governance priority, which requires international co-operation' (Wernli et al. 2017: 1). The policy discourses around AMR are also complex however, with Wernli et al. identifying five key policy frames that are evident in the debates around AMR, with each of these frames providing insights into AMR and the interdependencies between these policy frames: (i) 'AMR as a healthcare issue'; (ii) 'AMR as a development issue,' reflecting the burden of infectious diseases in low- and middle-income countries; (iii) the relationship between AMR and innovation, which recognises the importance of research and development for new antibiotics; (iv) AMR as a global health security issue; and (v) AMR and the role of a One-Health approach to addressing AMR (Wernli et al. 2017).

International cooperation will clearly play a key role in responding to AMR (Årdal et al. 2016). However, recent global health crises have revealed difficulties in ensuring effective responses to emerging public health crises, leaving the role of global health governance in leading responses to AMR unclear. The remainder of this chapter identifies four key areas that will present challenges for a global response to AMR: (i) the challenge of fitting responses to AMR within other global health governance frameworks that support urgent responses to health crises; (ii) the challenge of developing national and regional capacities to identify and respond to AMR; (iii) the challenge of developing common understandings and definitions of AMR; and finally (iv) the challenge of fitting AMR within the global priorities identified by the Sustainable Development Goals.

The International Health Regulations, Global Health Governance and AMR

Adopted to manage the international spread of infectious diseases, the International Health Regulations (2005) (IHR) (World Health Organization 2016a) could possibly provide a framework for improved surveillance and reporting of AMR. However, there has been debate over whether the scope of the IHR could include evolving events such as AMR or whether the IHR are more properly focused on emergency situations (Wernli et al. 2011; Kamradt-Scott 2011). It has been argued that AMR may, at least in some instances, fulfil two of the four IHR criteria for a 'public health emergency of international concern' (PHEIC) i.e. those relating to the seriousness of the public health impact of an event, and the potential for international spread of disease (Wernli et al. 2011: 3), with the remaining two IHR criteria being that the event is 'unusual or unexpected,' and that there is 'a significant risk of international travel or trade restrictions' (World Health Organization 2016a: Annex 2). It is certainly the case that the IHR provide a strong normative scaffold for the shared expectations about how both states and the international community should respond to the international spread of disease (Davies et al. 2015), as well as clear processes for reporting progress.

While patterns of AMR vary between countries (Review on Antimicrobial Resistance 2014), AMR certainly poses major risks to public health globally (World Health Organization 2015a). The focus of the IHR on managing global risks to public health, and the inclusion of consideration of whether there is 'a significant risk of international spread' as one of the criteria for determining whether events that may constitute a PHEIC should be notified to WHO (World Health Organization 2016a: Annex 2), provide a global perspective to the risks posed by spread of AMR. As it is now more than a decade since the revised IHR took effect in 2007, the IHR provide a familiar and well-established framework for the global community and, it has been argued that it may be possible to build on existing frameworks rather than building new ones (Wernli et al. 2011: 5). Yet these factors do not necessarily make the IHR an ideal mechanism for addressing AMR (Kamradt-Scott 2011), even though, with the global initiatives referred to above, global health governance seems set to play a key role in addressing AMR.

Despite the promise that initially heralded the adoption of the revised IHR in 2005 (Fidler and Gostin 2006), recent global health crises have revealed significant shortcomings in contemporary global health governance including, inadequate capacity building of national health systems, a failure by countries to comply with the IHR 2005 through the imposition of trade and travel restrictions contrary to WHO recommendations, and a lack of funding to support an effective global response to global public health emergencies (Gostin et al. 2015, 2016; Moon et al.

2015; Ottersen et al. 2016). Furthermore, the suitability of the IHR as a mechanism for addressing AMR remains unclear, with the primary focus of the IHR being on the global capacity to deal with global public health emergencies (Kamradt-Scott 2011). With the IHR's focus being on acute emergencies, rather than issues requiring sustained response over a prolonged period, their utility as a framework for coordinating global responses to AMR appears less certain (Wernli et al. 2017: 5; Kamradt-Scott 2011).

While a new treaty may provide a clear mechanism for addressing the challenges posed by AMR (Anomaly 2010; Hoffman, Outterson, Røttingen et al. 2015), as has been noted, 'Reaching such an ambitious legal agreement will take leadership, skill, and perseverance from a wide range of actors' (Rochford et al. 2018: 1977). A treaty would also need to balance stewardship of antibiotics and innovation with recognition of lack of access to antibiotics for many people, particularly in low and middle income countries (Padiyara et al. 2018: 3). Furthermore, as discussed below, the issue of capacity building remains an enduring challenge, particularly in low resource countries.

Building Capacity

A further difficulty associated with using the IHR as a mechanism for addressing AMR is in the challenges faced by many countries to meet their IHR core capacity requirements (Davies et al. 2015: 126-132; World Health Organization 2015b). The IHR require Member States to develop core capacities within their national health systems to 'detect, assess, notify and report events' that are within the scope of the IHR (Article 5). These national capacities required by the IHR will provide an important step in building surveillance capacities for AMR (Wernli et al. 2011). Countries were required to achieve the core capacity requirements of the IHR by 2012 i.e. within 5 years of the IHR coming into force, with some extensions possible, but many countries still had not achieved their core capacity requirements (World Health Organization 2016b). Although global collaboration (Goff et al. 2017) and regional networks may provide an additional mechanism for capacity building, particularly in developing regions (Bennett and Carney 2017), the challenge of building strong public health systems remains a key one for global health (Gostin et al. 2016; Moon et al. 2015).

In addition, although the World Health Assembly has urged its Member States to develop national action plans for antimicrobial resistance (World Health Assembly 2015), the results of 2013–2014 WHO survey showing that few countries reported having comprehensive national AMR plans (World Health Organization 2015c: 1), suggests that there may be considerable work to be done in many countries. More recently, a self-assessment survey of countries and their progress in developing and implementing national AMR plans also shows that considerable work remains, with only 60% of countries having a national multisectoral action plan on AMR, although a further 33% had plans in development (World Health Organization et al. 2018: 7). In addition, although 125 countries reported having awareness raising activities about AMR risks and human health, only 36 had campaigns in animal health (World Health Organization et al. 2018: 12). While 103 countries reported having a national surveillance system in humans, only 41 counties had systematic data collection in animals, and most countries have no surveillance system in place in the plant and environment sectors (World Health Organization et al. 2018: 15).

One key difficulty is that although the IHR require countries to develop their national capacities to deal with potential global public health emergencies that arise within their borders, poorer countries may have difficulty in finding the resources to support such capacity building (Gostin and Katz 2016: 276-277; Davies et al. 2015: 126-132), leaving many countries unable to achieve the capacities required by the IHR. There is renewed interest in developing sustainable mechanisms for global health financing, including financing of global public goods such as addressing antimicrobial resistance (Ottersen et al. 2017; Mendelson et al. 2016; Moon et al. 2017). Clearly there is a need for investment to address shared vulnerabilities in global health (Gostin 2017). Global commitments and the development of effective financing mechanisms will be key to the development of effective responses to AMR. Without them we may see a repeat of the difficulties in building IHR core capacities, with poorer countries lacking the resources to develop their national capacities.

Understandings and Definitions

Understandings of the mechanisms of development of AMR as well as definitions of key terms relating to infection and antimicrobial use are critical to effective policy response for AMR. Even the term 'antimicrobial resistance' may be poorly understood (Mendelson et al. 2017). The two pillars of the health policy response to antimicrobial resistance relate to control of its spread ('infection control') and to reduction of inappropriate antibiotic use that promotes it (antimicrobial stewardship) (Davies et al. 2013; Laxminarayan et al. 2013).

Measures of success and failure of public health policy are heavily contingent on definitions. The definition of 'inappropriate prescribing' remains poorly informed by research into antibiotic effects and is therefore regarded as a public policy research priority in the area of antibiotic resistance (Spellberg et al. 2011). Similarly, the definition of 'severe infection' or 'sepsis' is subject to major revision (Fullerton et al. 2017) and new definitions may alter the cohort included in this definition, especially at initial point of care where health policy must drive effective immediate responses (Fullerton et al. 2017).

These definitional questions are of key importance to policy initiatives such as antibiotic stewardship. AMR is an example of the tragedy of the commons in which overconsumption of a common resource harms the common good (Hollis and Maybarduk 2015; Giubilini and Savulescu 2020). For this reason, stewardship and the preservation of key antimicrobials is an important strategy in addressing AMR (Laxminarayan et al. 2013). Yet the development of policy responses for AMR is a particular challenge as there is a need to limit inappropriate use of antibiotics, (which assumes well-developed understandings of 'inappropriate prescribing'), while simultaneously ensuring equitable access to medicines (Laxminarayan et al. 2013, 2016; Padiyara et al. 2018; Selgelid 2007). An antibiotic that is harmful to the public health in terms of driving resistance in the longer term may be thought to have specific benefit to the individual for whom it is prescribed. This may lead to direct conflict between public health policy needs and the needs of an individual and means in turn that antimicrobial stewardship may be cast in a policing role.

These challenges may be described as ones of 'understandings' and of 'definitions.' To address these challenges additional funding is required to support research on the mechanisms for acquiring resistance to further our understandings of this important area. Agreed international standards for data collection on AMR (World Health Organization 2014) are also vital if surveillance is to be comprehensive and effective, making definitional issues ones of critical importance.

AMR and the Sustainable Development Goals (SDGs)

When the Sustainable Development Goals (SDGs) (United Nations 2015) were adopted by the United Nations General Assembly in September 2015, AMR was not listed amongst the 17 goals, although it is mentioned in the SDG declaration (World Health Organization 2015d: 103). Nor was there the inclusion of a broader SDG goal on global health security, which might have also provided a focus for action on AMR (Kickbusch et al. 2015). However, this is not to suggest that the SDGs will be irrelevant for global responses to AMR. For example, addressing antimicrobial resistance will clearly be important to achieving SDG3 ('Ensure healthy lives and promote well-being for all at all ages'), while the goal of universal health coverage in SDG3.8 will help to ensure the existence of strong health systems (Gostin 2017: 194). International trade of animals or products, the complexity of addressing both overconsumption and lack of access to medicines, and the relevance of trade agreements and intellectual property arrangements to research and development for new antimicrobials, all highlight the importance of considering the relevance of trade to the development of solutions to antimicrobial resistance (Hanefeld et al. 2017). Access to water and sanitation were also included as SDG6 (United Nations 2015). As the UK's Review on Antimicrobial Resistance has noted, improved water and sanitation can help to reduce antibiotic consumption by helping to prevent infections that may then be treated with antibiotics (Review on Antimicrobial Resistance 2016a: 21-23;

2016b). The association between poor sanitation, infections and antibiotic use shows that broader public health goals and improvements can play an important role in global strategies to prevent AMR (Review on Antimicrobial Resistance 2016a; 2016b).

Conclusion

Developing effective mechanisms to address the growing threat of AMR will be essential to safeguarding public health into the future. To achieve this will require, amongst other things, strong mechanisms for global health governance to support coordinated programs and building of capacity at the national, regional and global levels. The commitments to the development of national plans for AMR along with suggestions for new financing mechanisms to support capacity building and the funding of global public goods reflect a promising prioritisation of AMR. Whether we can develop practical and effective means of addressing AMR remains to be seen.

Acknowledgements Belinda Bennett gratefully acknowledges helpful discussions with Sara E Davies in the development of this chapter and Elizabeth Dallaston for her research assistance.

References

Adhikari, N.K.J., R.A. Fowler, S. Bhagwanjee, and G.D. Rubenfeld. 2010. Critical care and the global burden of critical illness in adults. *The Lancet* 375: 1339–1346.

Anomaly, J. 2010. Combating resistance: The case for a global antibiotics treaty. *Public Health Ethics* 3 (1): 13–22.

Årdal, C., K. Outterson, S.J. Hoffman, A. Ghafur, M. Sharland, N. Ranganathan, et al. 2016. International cooperation to improve access to and sustain effectiveness of antimicrobials. *Lancet* 387: 296–307.

Bennett, B., and T. Carney. 2017. Public health emergencies of international concern: Global, regional and local responses to risk. *Medical Law Review* 25 (2): 223–239.

Davies, S.C., T. Fowler, J. Watson, D.M. Livermore, and D. Walker. 2013. Annual report of the Chief Medical Officer: Infection and the rise of antimicrobial resistance. *Lancet* 381 (9878): 1606–1609.

Davies, S.E., A. Kamradt-Scott, and S. Rushton. 2015. *Disease diplomacy: International norms and global health security*. Baltimore: Johns Hopkins University Press.

Fidler, D.P., and L.O. Gostin. 2006. The new International Health Regulations: An historic development for international law and public health. *Journal of Law, Medicine & Ethics*. 34: 85–94.

Fullerton, J.N., K. Thompson, A. Shetty, J.R. Iredell, et al. 2017. New sepsis definition changes incidence of sepsis in the intensive care unit. *Critical Care and Resuscitation*. 19 (1): 9–13.

Giubilini, A. and J. Savulescu. 2020. Moral responsibility and the justification of policies to preserve antimicrobial effectiveness. In *Ethics and drug resistance: Collective responsibility for global public health*, ed. E. Jamrozik and M. Selgelid. Cham: Springer.

Goff, D.A., R. Kullar, E.J. Goldstein, M. Gilchrist, D. Nathwani, A.C. Cheng, et al. 2017. A global call from five countries to collaborate in antibiotic stewardship: United we succeed, divided we might fail. *Lancet Infectious Diseases* 17: e56–e63.

Gostin, L.O. 2017. Our shared vulnerability to dangerous pathogens. *Medical Law Review* 25 (2): 185–199.

Gostin, L.O., and R. Katz. 2016. The International Health Regulations: The governing framework for global health security. *The Milbank Quarterly* 94 (2): 264–313.

Gostin, L.O., M. DeBartolo, and E. Friedman. 2015. The International Health Regulations 10 years on: The governing framework for global health security. *Lancet* 386: 2222–2226.

Gostin, L.O., O. Tomori, S. Wibulpolprasert, A.K. Jha, J. Frenk, S. Moon, et al. 2016. Toward a common secure future: Four global commissions in the wake of Ebola. *PLoS Medicine* 13 (5): e1002042. https://doi.org/10.1371/journal.pmed.1002042.

Hanefeld, J., M. Khan, G. Tomson, and R. Smith. 2017. Trade is central to achieving the Sustainable Development Goals: A case study of antimicrobial resistance. *BMJ* 358: j3505. https://doi.org/10.1136/bmj.j3505.

Ho, C.W.L., and T.-L. Lee. 2020. Global governance of antimicrobial resistance: A legal and regulatory toolkit. In *Ethics and drug resistance: Collective responsibility for global public health*, ed. E. Jamrozik and M. Selgelid. Cham: Springer.

Hoffman, S., K. Outterson, J.-A. Røttingen, O. Cars, C. Clift, Z. Rizvi, et al. 2015. Editorial: An international legal framework to address antimicrobial resistance. *Bulletin of the World Health Organization* 93: 66.

Hoffman, S.J., J.-A. Røttingen, and J. Frenk. 2015. International law has a role to play in addressing antibiotic resistance. *Journal of Law, Medicine & Ethics* 43 (3 Suppl): 65–67.

Hoffman, S.J., G.M. Caleo, N. Daulaire, S. Elbe, P. Matsoso, E. Mossialos, et al. 2015. Strategies for achieving global collective action on antimicrobial resistance. *Bulletin of the World Health Organization* 93: 867–876.

Hollis, A., and P. Maybarduk. 2015. Antibiotic resistance is a tragedy of the commons that necessitates global cooperation. *Journal of Law, Medicine & Ethics* 43 (3 Suppl): 33–37.

Howard, S.J., M. Catchpole, J. Watson, and S.C. Davies. 2013. Antibiotic resistance: Global response needed. *Lancet Infectious Diseases* 13 (12): 1001–1003.

Kamradt-Scott, A. 2011. A public health emergency of international concern? Response to a proposal to apply the International Health Regulations to antimicrobial resistance. *PLoS Medicine* 8 (4): e1001021.

Kickbusch, I., J. Orbinski, T. Winkler, and A. Schnabel. 2015. We need a sustainable development goal 18 on global health security. *Lancet* 385: 1069.

Laxminarayan, R., A. Duse, C. Wattal, A. Zaidi, H. Wertheim, N. Sumpradit, et al. 2013. Antibiotic resistance – The need for global solutions. *Lancet Infectious Diseases* 13: 1057–1098.

Laxminarayan, R., P. Matsoso, S. Pant, C. Brower, J.-A. Røttingen, K. Klugman, et al. 2016. Access to effective antimicrobials: A worldwide challenge. *Lancet* 387: 168–175.

Littman, J., A.M. Viens, and D.S. Silva. 2020. The super-wicked problem of antimicrobial resistance. In *Ethics and drug resistance: Collective responsibility for global public health*, ed. E. Jamrozik and M. Selgelid. Cham: Springer.

Mendelson, M., O. Dar, S.J. Hoffman, R. Laxminarayan, M.M. Mpundu, and J.-A. Røttingen. 2016. A global antimicrobial conservation fund for low- and middle-income countries. *International Journal of Infectious Diseases* 51: 70–72.

Mendelson, M., M. Balasegaram, T. Jinks, C. Pulcini, and M. Sharland. 2017. Antibiotic resistance has a language problem. *Nature* 545: 23–25.

Moon, S., D. Sridhar, M.A. Pate, A.K. Jha, et al. 2015. Will Ebola change the game? Ten essential reforms before the next pandemic. The report of the Harvard-LSHTM independent panel on the global response to Ebola. *Lancet* 386: 2204–2221.

Moon, S., J.-A. Røttingen, and J. Frenk. 2017. Global public goods for health: Weaknesses and opportunities in the global health system. *Health Economics, Policy and Law* 12: 195–205.

Ottersen, T., S.J. Hoffman, and G. Groux. 2016. Ebola again shows the International Health Regulations are broken: What can be done differently to prepare for the next epidemic? *American Journal of Law & Medicine* 42: 356–392.

Ottersen, T., R. Elovainio, D.B. Evans, D. McCoy, D. McIntyre, F. Meheus, et al. 2017. Towards a coherent global framework for health financing: Recommendations and recent developments. *Health Economics, Policy and Law* 12: 285–296.

Padiyara, P., H. Inoue, and M. Sprenger. 2018. Global governance mechanisms to address antimicrobial resistance. *Infectious Diseases: Research and Treatment* 11: 1–4.

Piddock, L.J. 2012. The crisis of no new antibiotics – What is the way forward? *Lancet Infectious Diseases* 12 (3): 249–253.

Review on Antimicrobial Resistance. 2014. *Antimicrobial resistance: Tackling a crisis for the health and wealth of nations*. London.

———. 2015. *Tackling a global health crisis: Initial steps*. London.

———. 2016a. *Tackling drug-resistant infections globally: Final report and recommendations*. London.

———. 2016b. *Infection prevention, control and surveillance: Limiting the development and spread of drug resistance*. London.

Rochford, C., D. Sridhar, N. Woods, et al. 2018. Global governance of antimicrobial resistance. *Lancet* 391: 1976–1978.

Selgelid, M.J. 2007. Ethics and drug resistance. *Bioethics* 21 (4): 218–229.

Seymour, C.W., T.D. Rea, J.M. Kahn, A.J. Walkey, D.M. Yealy, and D.C. Angus. 2012. Severe sepsis in pre-hospital emergency care: Analysis of incidence, care, and outcome. *American Journal of Respiratory and Critical Care Medicine*. 186 (12): 1264–1271.

Spellberg, B., R. Guidos, D. Gilbert, J. Bradley, H.W. Boucher, W.M. Scheld, et al. 2008. The epidemic of antibiotic-resistant infections: A call to action for the medical community from the Infectious Diseases Society of America. *Clinical Infectious Diseases* 46 (2): 155–164.

Spellberg, B., M. Blaser, R.J. Guidos, H.W. Boucher, J.S. Bradley, B.I. Eisenstein, et al. 2011. Combating antimicrobial resistance: Policy recommendations to save lives. *Clinical Infectious Diseases* 52 (Suppl 5): S397–S428.

United Nations. 2015. *Sustainable Development Goals*. Available from: www.un.org/sustainabledevelopment/sustainable-development-goals.

United Nations General Assembly. 2016. *Political declaration of the high-level meeting of the General Assembly on antimicrobial resistance* (A/RES/71/3).

Viens, A.M., and J. Littman. 2015. Is antimicrobial resistance a slowly emerging disaster? *Public Health Ethics*. 8(3): 255-265.

Vincent, J.L., J. Rello, J. Marshall, E. Silva, A. Anzueto, C.D. Martin, et al. 2009. International study of the prevalence and outcomes of infection in intensive care units. *JAMA* 302 (21): 2323–2329.

Wernli, D., T. Haustein, J. Conly, Y. Carmeli, I. Kickbusch, and S. Harbarth. 2011. A call for action: The application of the International Health Regulations to the global threat of antimicrobial resistance. *PLoS Medicine* 8 (4): e1001022.

Wernli, D., P.S. Jørgensen, C.M. Morel, S. Carroll, S. Harbarth, N. Levrat, et al. 2017. Mapping global policy discourse on antimicrobial resistance. *BMJ Global Health* 2: e000378.

Woolhouse, M., and J. Farrar. 2014. An intergovernmental panel on antimicrobial resistance. *Nature* 509: 555–557.

World Health Assembly. 2014. *Antimicrobial resistance* (WHA67.25).

———. 2015. *Resolution WHA68.7 – Global action plan on antimicrobial resistance.*

World Health Organization. 2014. *Antimicrobial resistance: Global report on surveillance.* Geneva: World Health Organization.

———. 2015a. *Global action plan on antimicrobial resistance*. Geneva: World Health Organization.

———. 2015b. *Implementation of the International Health Regulations (2005): Report of the Review Committee on second extensions for establishing national public health capacities and on IHR implementation* (A68/22 Add.1).

———. 2015c. *Worldwide country situation analysis: Response to antimicrobial resistance.* Geneva: World Health Organization.

———. 2015d. *Health in 2015: From MDGs Millennium Development Goals to SDGs Sustainable Development Goals*. Geneva: World Health Organization.

———. 2016a. *International Health Regulations (2005)*. 3rd ed. Geneva.

———. 2016b. *Implementation of the International Health Regulations (2005): Annual report on the implementation of the International Health Regulations (2005). Report by the Director-General* (WHA A69/20).

World Health Organization, Food and Agricultural Organization of the United Nations, World Organisation for Animal Health. 2018. *Monitoring global progress on addressing antimicrobial resistance: Analysis report of the second round of results of AMR country self-assessment survey 2018.*

6

Tackling Anti-microbial Resistance: An Ethical Framework for Rational Antibiotic Use

Jasper Littmann, Annette Rid, and Alena Buyx

Abstract To reduce the effect of antimicrobial resistance and preserve antibiotic effectiveness, clinical practice guidelines and health policy documents call for the "rational use" of antibiotics that aims to avoid unnecessary or minimally effective antibiotic prescriptions. In this paper, we show that rational use programmes can lead to ethical conflicts because they place some patients at risk of harm – for example, a delayed switch to second-line antibiotics for community-acquired pneumonia is associated with increased fatality rates. Implementing the rational use of antibiotics can therefore lead to conflicts between promoting patients' clinical interests and preserving antibiotic effectiveness for future use. The resulting ethical dilemma for clinicians, patients and policy makers has so far not been adequately addressed. We argue that existing guidance for acceptable risks in clinical research can help to define risk thresholds for the rational use of antibiotics. We develop an ethical framework that allows clinicians and policy-makers to evaluate policies for rational antibiotic use in six practical steps.

This paper is an extended version of: Littmann J, Rid A, Buyx A: Tackling anti-microbial resistance: ethical framework for rational antibiotic use. European Journal of Public Health 2018; 28(2): 359–363. A fuller defense of our framework is provided in: Rid A, Littmann J, Buyx A: Evaluating the risks of public health programs: rational antibiotic use and antimicrobial resistance. Bioethics 2019; 33(7): 734-748.

J. Littmann
National Institute of Public Health, Centre for Antimicrobial Resistance, Oslo, Norway

Institute for Ethics and History of Medicine, Technical University, Munich, Germany

A. Rid
Department of Bioethics, The Clinical Center, National Institutes of Health, Bethesda, MD, USA

A. Buyx (✉)
Institute for Ethics and History of Medicine, Technical University, Munich, Germany
e-mail: a.buyx@tum.de

Keywords Antimicrobial resistance · Medical ethics · Rational use of antibiotics · Research ethics · Rationing · Acceptable risk

Introduction

Antimicrobial resistance (AMR) has been described as one of the major threats to public health in the twenty-first century and sparked concerns about the possibility of a post-antibiotic era, in which many infections are no longer treatable (WHO 2014; General Assembly of the United Nations 2016; Davies et al. 2013). Such a development would not only have detrimental effects on patient care, but is also likely to significantly affect public health, agriculture, as well as economic and national security (PCAST 2014; O'Neill 2014; Adeyi et al. 2017; OECD 2018).

Over the past few years, the challenge of AMR has increasingly been recognised by policy makers. The World Health Organization (WHO) developed a global action plan on AMR (WHO 2011, 2015), the United Nations General Assembly passed a declaration on the issue (General Assembly of the United Nations 2016) and the G20—a forum of the world's major economies—has placed AMR on its agenda (Bundesministerium für Gesundheit 2011). In addition, considerable investments have been made to strengthen and incentivise the development of new antibiotics (Boucher et al. 2013; Drive-AB-12 2018; Rex 2014; Outterson et al. 2016a, b).

Since one of the major causes of AMR is the overprescription and overconsumption of antibiotics, comprehensive response plans to preserve antibiotic effectiveness do not focus solely on the development of new drugs. They also include a wide range of measures, including surveillance, infection control and, crucially, the promotion of the "rational" use of antibiotics (WHO 2014). Rational use programmes primarily focus on avoiding unnecessary prescriptions of antibiotic treatments, for example in the context of viral respiratory infections. However, they also include practices that involve delaying or withholding access to antibiotics that are known to be beneficial. These practices can place some patients at risk of harm and thereby lead to conflicts between two important ethical goals: promoting patients' clinical interests and preserving antibiotic effectiveness for future use.

The ethical conflict between these goals has so far not been adequately addressed. In this paper, we describe programmes for rational antibiotic use and show when they require placing some patients at risk of harm for the benefit of managing the existing pool of effective antibiotics. We argue that ethical guidance on acceptable risks in clinical research can help to develop acceptable programmes for rational antibiotic use. Based on a recognized ethical framework for risk and risk-benefit evaluations in clinical research, we propose a novel framework that allows clinicians and policy-makers to evaluate when rational antibiotic use is (or is not) ethically justified.

Rational Use of Antibiotics

The promotion of "rational" antibiotic use – sometimes referred to as "prudent" or "appropriate" use – is a key component of many response plans to AMR (Bundesministerium für Gesundheit 2011; UK Department of Health 2013; Public Health Agency of Canada 2014; The White House 2014; Australian Department for Health 2015). The WHO provided the most widely cited definition of the rational use of medicines in general, which includes the rational use of antibiotics. According to WHO, this requires that "patients receive medications appropriate to their clinical need, in doses that meet their own individual requirements, for an adequate period of time, and at the lowest cost to them and their community" (WHO 1985). Elsewhere, the WHO defined appropriate antibiotic use as the "cost-effective use of antimicrobials which maximizes clinical therapeutic effect while minimizing drug-related toxicity and the development of antimicrobial resistance" (WHO 2011). Most concise is the definition provided by the Alliance for the Prudent Use of Antibiotics (APUA), which defines prudent use as "the right drug for the right condition for the right amount of time" (Wilson and Tan 2010).

Notwithstanding some differences in meaning, these definitions all delineate types of antibiotic use that are clearly "irrational"—that is, obvious instances of overuse or misuse where antibiotics are prescribed or taken even though they are not the appropriate treatment. For example, antibiotics are an appropriate treatment for "strep throat", which is caused by a bacterium susceptible to certain antibiotics. However, they are not an appropriate treatment for most sore throats, which are caused by viruses against which antibiotics are not effective.

There is a wide array of interventions designed to reduce antibiotic prescribing, and evidence suggests that restrictive measures, which limit the availability of antibiotics, have a higher chance of success than information campaigns or educational interventions that teach prescribing clinicians about AMR (Charani et al. 2011; Davey et al. 2013). In many instances, such restrictions appear to be a promising and effective way of reducing antibiotic use. For instance, recent research has shown that antibiotic prescribing in primary care can be restricted substantially, without a negative effect on clinical outcomes, through a practice called delayed prescribing (Schuetz et al. 2009; Spurling et al. 2013; Little et al. 2014). Here patients for whom antibiotics are unlikely to be an appropriate treatment—say most patients with sore throats—receive a prescription that they can use at the pharmacy if their symptoms do not improve on their own within a few days. Receiving such a prescription gives patients reassurance, even though only few end up filling it. A Cochrane review concluded that delayed prescribing offers no additional risks to the patient, while offering similar patient satisfaction when compared to immediate prescribing (Spurling et al. 2013).

So understood, rational use of antibiotics is ethically justified because it promotes patients' clinical interests while also preserving antibiotic effectiveness for future use. Not only are present patients spared the side effects of unnecessary treatment, avoiding such treatment also curbs the spread of antibiotic resistance and thereby helps to ensure that existing antibiotics remain effective to treat future patients. Indeed, because rational use so understood promotes the interests of present as well as future patients, clinicians and policy-makers are ethically required to ensure that patients use "the right drug for the right condition for the right amount of time" (Wilson and Tan 2010).

Ethically Challenging Instances of Rational Use

In addition to avoiding unnecessary antibiotic use, rational use programmes embrace practices that restrict access to antibiotics even when treatment would reduce a given patient's health risk (Millar 2012). One example for this are programmes that ask clinicians to factor resistance thresholds in the community when they suggest antibiotic treatment to their patients. For example, clinical practice guidelines for treating community-acquired pneumonia recommend the use of macrolides—a particular class of antibiotics—unless 25% or more of the relevant pathogens are resistant to macrolides in the given local community (Mandell et al. 2007). Only then should clinicians switch to more effective second-line drugs (Mandell et al. 2007).[1] When considering the entire patient population, this is a sensible recommendation, since it is to be expected that macrolides—the first line of treatment—remains effective in most patients if resistance is below 25%. However, a delayed switch to second-line drugs negatively affects clinical outcomes in some patients, notably those with severe pneumonia. Some authors estimate that a similar guideline has carried a mortality risk of more than 1% for all patients in the past (Daneman et al. 2008). Rational use practices of this type effectively delay or withhold a proven beneficial antibiotic in order to curb the spread of antimicrobial resistance. This places some present patients at risk for the sake of future patients.

In these and comparable cases, the rational use of antibiotics confronts clinicians with a trade-off between promoting their present patients' best clinical interests and helping to maintain effective antibiotic treatments for future patients (Kollef and Micek 2014). This trade-off seems particularly stark for several reasons (Littmann et al. 2015; Littmann and Buyx 2018). First, it is difficult to measure the contribution of any individual course of antibiotics to the emergence of AMR in a population, so that estimates about the benefits of rational use programmes are relatively uncertain. It seems likely, however, that delaying or withholding any given antibiotic treatment makes no more than a very small contribution to curbing AMR and, in some cases, no contribution at all. For example, a patient might develop resistant

[1] Since the time of writing, an updated version of the consensus guidelines has superseded the cited work (Metlay et al. 2019).

bacteria but die before transmitting these to other people or the environment. As a result, rational use programmes that involve delaying or withholding antibiotic treatment are neither necessary nor sufficient for addressing AMR. Moreover, the benefits of preserving antibiotics may accrue to unknown people in the potentially distant future. By contrast, the benefits of antibiotic treatment for the present patient are much easier to measure and can therefore be predicted with greater certainty. Antibiotic treatment also has immediate benefits that accrue to known or "identified" persons. These differences readily explain why a typical clinician who is tasked with delaying or withholding antibiotics from her present patients with the goal of tackling AMR would feel an acute ethical conflict (Cohen et al. 2015).

Bioethicists have started to discuss this ethical conflict (Selgelid 2007; Battin et al. 2009; Millar 2012; Oczkowski 2017; Littmann and Buyx 2014; Littmann et al. 2015). However, at both the clinical and policy level, there is no ethical guidance on when rational use programmes that involve delaying or withholding antibiotics and hence compromise the best clinical interests of present patients are acceptable. Moreover, many policy documents lack explicit discussion of any ethical challenges, and those that include ethical considerations are narrowly disease- and pathogen-specific (Bundesministerium für Gesundheit 2011; WHO 2011; Davies et al. 2013; Andreasen 2014). What is therefore needed is a more specific analysis of whether and when it is acceptable to restrict antibiotics use with the goal of curbing AMR, even when doing so poses risks to present patients and thereby compromises their best clinical interests.

The Analogy to Clinical Research

To address this question, it is helpful to consider more generally whether and when it is justified for clinicians not to promote the best clinical interests of their present patient. Standard professional guidance takes a relatively restrictive stance on this issue. For example, the World Medical Association states that clinicians owe their patients "complete loyalty", and that they may place the interests of others above those of the patient only in "exceptional situations" (Williams 2015). However, closer analysis reveals many clinical practices that place the interests of other patients, individuals or society above the interests of a given present patient (Wendler 2010). Consider, for example, that clinicians routinely give vaccinations not to protect the present patient, but to maintain herd immunity; that clinicians transplant kidneys from healthy individuals to patients with renal failure in order to enable these patients to live a better and longer life; and that clinicians allow younger colleagues to gain experience and perform procedures for the first time, even though they know that this will result in higher complication rates for the present patient. Importantly, these practices are not only frequent, but ethically justified provided that a number of conditions are met (Wendler 2010). This finding raises the possibility of evaluating the ethical acceptability of rational use programmes for antibiotics in comparison to other practices that involve compromising the interests of individual patients for the benefit of others.

For such comparisons to be both sound and useful, it is essential to identify comparator practices that are relevantly similar to rational use programmes for antibiotics and widely considered to be acceptable (Sunstein 1993). Moreover, detailed ethical guidance on how to evaluate the given comparator practice should ideally exist. Clinical research fulfils all three desiderata, as the following paragraphs demonstrate.

Clinical research is a subset of research with human participants that focuses on evaluating methods to prevent, treat or cure illness and disease, or on generating the knowledge necessary to develop such methods. One of the key characteristics of clinical research is that investigators expose participants to some risks for the potential benefits of unknown patients in the potentially distant future. Clinician-investigators routinely perform research procedures that do not promote the best clinical interests of the present patient-participant, but serve solely to address research questions. In fact, the majority of clinical trials involve procedures that have no prospect of clinical benefit for participants but help to answer important research questions. For example, most clinical trials involve additional blood draws, biopsies or imaging procedures that would not be performed as part of routine clinical care, but serve to test the safety and efficacy of an investigational drug. Moreover, phase 1 trials with healthy individuals by definition have no prospect of clinical benefit. It is widely considered acceptable for clinician-investigators to perform these "net risk" procedures and trials—and thereby deviate from the general clinical norm of promoting the present patient's best clinical interests—because clinical research generates knowledge with the potential to improve the health or care of future patients (WMA 2013; CIOMS 2016). That is, the potential benefits of clinical research for future populations are widely considered to justify that investigators expose patient-participants to some level of net research risk.

Importantly, the potential benefits for future patients—or the so-called "social value" of the research—is generally seen as the fundamental justification for exposing participants to net research risks, not the participants' informed consent. Participants' consent is, of course, relevant for determining what levels of net research risk are acceptable in socially valuable research. Only small levels of net risk are acceptable when participants cannot give their own informed consent, for example in research involving children, or when obtaining participants' consent is not feasible, for example in research on large datasets that were originally collected for clinical (and not for research) purposes. By contrast, greater net risks are acceptable when participants give their voluntary and informed consent. However, it is generally accepted—and for good reason in our view—that research without social value is not justified even when the research poses low net risks and participants consent (Wendler and Rid 2017). This underscores that the fundamental justification for exposing participants to net research risks lies in the potential benefits of clinical research for future patients.

Restricting antibiotic use with the goal of curbing AMR is relevantly similar to clinical research in this important respect. Just like in research, clinicians expose the present patient to some risks of harm for the potential benefits of unknown patients in the potentially distant future. Moreover, what level of risk is acceptable arguably depends on whether the present patient consents to delaying or foregoing antibiotic treatment that would be in her best clinical interests. In clinical research, it is not certain that any given clinical trial generates findings that make a significant contribution to improving the health or care of future patients and populations. Moreover, the enrolment of any single patient-participant is uncertain to make a significant difference to the value of any given trial. Yet without sufficient overall participation, trials—and clinical research more generally—would fail. Rational use programmes that involve delaying or withholding antibiotics are similar in this respect. It is not only uncertain that such programmes will make a significant contribution to addressing AMR, but restricting a single patient's access to antibiotics may not lead to a measurable effect on the overall level of AMR. Yet reducing antibiotic prescriptions overall is a key component of strategies for curbing AMR and ensuring that bacterial infections can still be treated effectively in the future (Costelloe et al. 2010; Davies et al. 2013). Given this relevant similarity between clinical research and rational use programmes that delay or withhold antibiotics, and considering that it is widely accepted for clinician-investigators to impose some level of net risk on patient-participants for the potential benefit of future patients (Selgelid 2007; Kollef and Micek 2014), it should also be acceptable to impose comparable levels of risks on patients in order to preserve antibiotic effectiveness for future patients.[2]

Moreover, there is a long-standing and nuanced debate about acceptable risk in clinical research. This does not only mean that our judgments about acceptable risks are relatively considered in the research context, but also that detailed ethical guidance in this area exists (WMA 2013; CIOMS 2016; Emanuel et al. 2008). Clinical research therefore fulfils the three desiderata for sound and helpful comparisons formulated above: it is relevantly similar to rational use programmes that delay or withhold antibiotics for the sake of curbing AMR; it is widely considered an acceptable exception from the general principle that clinicians should act in the best interests of the present patient; and detailed ethical guidance on how to evaluate research risks, including net research risks, exists. This suggests that judgments about acceptable risk in clinical research can inform the ethical evaluation of rational use programmes that impose risks on present patients with the goal of curbing AMR and safeguarding antibiotic effectiveness for future patients (Rid et al. 2019).

An Ethical Framework for Evaluating Rational Antibiotic Use

For clinician-researchers to justifiably impose risks on patient-participants in clinical research, a number of conditions must be met. Specifically, the research must be scientifically valid and socially valuable; the risks to participants have to be

[2] There are, of course, relevant dissimilarities between clinical research and rational use programmes that involve delaying or withholding antibiotics. However, as we argue elsewhere in more detail, the similarities between the two clearly dominate the dissimilarities (Rid et al. 2019).

minimised and reasonable in relation to the potential clinical benefits for them and/or the social value of the research; and, when participants cannot or do not consent, any net risks to them should be no greater than minimal or, in cases of compelling social value, no greater than a minor increase over minimal risk (WMA 2013; CIOMS 2016).

To operationalise these conditions, one of the authors of this paper (AR) has developed a systematic framework for evaluating research risks and potential benefits based on prominent research ethics guidelines and literature (Rid and Wendler 2011). This framework can be usefully adapted to evaluate the risks of rational use programmes that involve delaying or withholding antibiotics from patients who could clinically benefit (Appendix). The framework is most useful for evaluating rational use programmes that do not require clinicians to obtain the patient's informed consent for restricting antibiotics. In particular, the minimal risk threshold for research without informed consent (Rid 2014) provides much needed orientation regarding acceptable levels of unconsented to net risks in the public health context. However, the framework could also help to evaluate rational use programmes that would require the patient's informed consent. Here, the debate about upper net risk limits in research with competent consenting adults is particularly informative (London 2006; Miller and Joffe 2009).

The framework sets out six steps for evaluating rational use programmes that involve delaying or withholding antibiotics. A hypothetical programme to restrict antibiotic use for lower respiratory tract infections (LRTIs) helps to illustrate how these steps would work in practice (Table 20.1, Ethical framework for rational antibiotic use).

The first step—*ensure and enhance the programme's social value*—requires decision-makers to develop rational use programmes based on sound evidence and policy methods. This is to ensure that all programmes are rigorously developed and judged to be both feasible and effective. For example, the available data should suggest that delaying or withholding the given antibiotics for LRTIs has the potential to help curb AMR. Data should also be sufficient to estimate the risks of restricting the antibiotics for patients; if there is too much uncertainty regarding how likely patients will suffer harm, relevant data should first be gathered in a research study. For programmes that meet these conditions, step one also requires conducting (and/or reviewing) observational research on their implementation. For example, how does restricted antibiotics use for LRTIs affect prescription rates, clinical outcomes, and antimicrobial resistance in the community? Such research serves to confirm that the given programme is indeed effective, while also expanding the existing knowledge of AMR. Evidence from accompanying observational research should inform regular re-evaluations of the programme.

The second step—*identify the programme interventions*—requires considering how the care of patients under the given rational use programme would differ from recommended standard care. Of course, the key difference would be that antibiotics are delayed or withheld under clearly specified circumstances. However, programmes might also include supplementary, non-routine interventions that aim to reduce the risks of restricting antibiotic use. Importantly, these non-routine

Table Ethical framework for rational antibiotic use

Step	Elements	Example
1. Ensure and enhance the policy's social value	1. Ensure that restricting antibiotics use for the given condition is based on sound evidence and policy methods	Available data allow estimating the clinical and public health impact of restricted antibiotics use for lower respiratory tract infections
		Policy to restrict antibiotics use for lower respiratory tract infections is rigorously developed (policy analysis, stakeholder consultation, etc.) and judged to be feasible and effective
	2. Ensure that restricting antibiotics use for the given condition passes a minimum threshold of social value	Restricted antibiotics use for lower respiratory tract infections has the potential to address antimicrobial resistance, a major public health problem
	3. Enhance the knowledge to be gained from the policy and use it to refine the policy	Initiate research[a] to evaluate how restricted antibiotics use for lower respiratory tract infections affects prescription rates, clinical outcomes, antimicrobial resistance etc. and update policy as new evidence comes in
		Evaluate how the experience with restricting antibiotics use for lower respiratory tract infections can inform the management of antibiotics use for other conditions (e.g. urinary tract infection)
2. Identify the policy interventions	1. Identify the policy intervention and any supplementary (non-routine) interventions to protect patients	Policy intervention: restricted antibiotics use for lower respiratory tract infections
		Supplementary interventions: provide relevant information to patients in writing (e.g. signs of worsening condition, next steps in this situation), provide 1-time respiratory therapy session to manage symptoms
		Exclude routine clinical interventions from analysis: provide relevant information verbally, provide supportive measures for lower respiratory tract infections (e.g. mucolytics, inhalation, pain medication)
	2. Ensure that each supplementary intervention is essential for protecting patients	Could consider whether written patient information is essential

(continued)

Table (continued)

Step	Elements	Example
3. Evaluate and reduce the risks to patients	1. Evaluate the risks of the policy intervention and each supplementary intervention	Restricting antibiotics use for lower respiratory tract infections poses risks (e.g. of increased complications such as pneumonia or empyema), which may require antibiotics and/or hospitalisation)
		Providing relevant information to patients in writing (rather than verbally) can cause mild anxiety
	2. Reasonably reduce the risks	Ensure that routine clinical interventions to treat lower respiratory tract infections are implemented (e.g. supportive measures)
		Ensure that serious harms, should they occur, are adequately managed at no financial cost to the patient (e.g. antibiotics and/or hospitalisation) and patients receive compensation for any lasting serious harms
		Actively monitor or exclude patient groups from policy who are at increased risk of complications or other serious harms (e.g. immunodeficiency)
		Instruct clinicians to exercise judgment in individual cases
		Reassure patients about written information sheet
4. Evaluate and enhance the potential benefits for patients	1. Evaluate the potential clinical benefits of the policy intervention and each supplementary intervention	Restricting antibiotics use for lower respiratory tract infections spares patients the risks of treatment (e.g. diarrhea) 1-time respiratory therapy session helps to manage symptoms
	2. Enhance the potential clinical benefits	Consider complementing 1-time respiratory therapy session with educational material
5. Evaluate whether the interventions pose net risks	1. Determine whether the risks of each individual intervention exceed the intervention's potential clinical benefits (implies net risks): Would an *informed clinician* who is committed solely to promoting the patient's clinical interests recommend the intervention?	*Informed clinician* would not recommend withholding antibiotic treatment for lower respiratory tract infections or measures to manage the resulting risks (e.g. written information, active monitoring): net risks
		Informed clinician would recommend respiratory therapy session: no net risks
	2. Determine whether the unit of policy and supplementary interventions pose net risks: would an *informed clinician* recommend the unit of interventions?	*Informed clinician* would not recommend unit of interventions: potential clinical benefits of respiratory therapy session do not outweigh the risks of withholding antibiotic treatment and measures to manage the resulting risks

(continued)

Table (continued)

Step	Elements	Example
6. Evaluate whether the net risks are justified by the policy's social value	1. Determine the level of cumulative net risk posed to patients	Relatively small level of net risk from withholding antibiotic treatment and measures to manage the resulting risks
	2. Determine whether the policy's cumulative net risks fall within the general range of acceptable net risk: could judge in light of net risk limits in biomedical research, notably the "minimal risk"" threshold in research without informed consent for rational use programmes that do not require clinicians to obtain the patient's informed consent and upper net risk limits in research for rational use programmes that require informed consent	Net risks from withholding antibiotic treatment for lower respiratory tract infections arguably falls within the range of acceptable net risk in clinical research (i.e. the net risks arguably fall below the minimal risk threshold)
	3. Evaluate whether the given level of cumulative net risk is proportionate to the social value of implementing the policy: would an *ideal social arbiter* recommend the policy?	*Ideal social arbiter* may recommend the policy, given the importance of curbing antimicrobial resistance and the arguably minimal net risks to patients

The framework is adapted from an existing framework for risk-benefit evaluations in biomedical research (Rid and Wendler 2011; see Appendix for additional details). Example: hypothetical policy to restrict antibiotics use (delayed or no prescription) for lower respiratory tract infections without obtaining the patients' informed consent

[a]Research to evaluate the impact of restricted antibiotics use for a given condition has to be judged based on standard ethical criteria for research (CIOMS 2016; WMA 2013)

interventions can carry their own risks. For example, if antibiotics for LRTIs were delayed or withheld, patients might be informed about signs of pneumonia or empyema (i.e. potential more serious complications of an initial infection) in writing, rather than verbally as in standard practice, so as to ensure that they know when to seek expert advice and thereby reduce risks to them. However, receiving written information can itself cause concern among patients. It is therefore essential to identify all programme interventions in order to comprehensively evaluate the risks that the given rational use programme poses to patients. As part of this step, the need for any supplementary interventions should also be scrutinized with a view to avoiding unnecessary risks. For example, do patients really require written information?

Step three—*evaluate and reduce the risks to patients*—requires evaluating the risks of all programme interventions, including those of any supplementary interventions, based on the available evidence. Moreover, all reasonable measures must be taken to reduce the risks to patients. For example, if written information about pneumonia and/or empyema is considered necessary, how can this information be conveyed in ways that reduce anxiety and stress for patients? Similarly, rational use programmes that involve delaying or withholding antibiotics need to ensure that patients who suffer serious harms are adequately treated at no financial cost. In the case of restricting antibiotics for LRTIs, for instance, it must be guaranteed that any collections of pus in the pleural cavity (i.e. empyemas) are promptly treated for free. Patients with any lasting serious harms should also receive compensation. Furthermore, patient groups at increased risk of experiencing serious harm—for example, patients with immune deficiency—should either be actively monitored or excluded from the programme. Guidelines should also instruct clinicians to exercise their judgment in individual cases.

Step four—*evaluate and enhance the potential benefits for patients*—requires evaluating based on the available evidence to what extent patients could benefit clinically from the given rational use programme. For example, not receiving antibiotics for LRTIs means avoiding their side effects and reducing the risk of infection with *Clostridium difficile*—which is associated with antibiotic use and sometimes leads to a life-threatening infection of the colon—or resistant infection in future. Moreover, non-routine supplementary interventions can have potential clinical benefits for patients. For instance, if a one-time respiratory therapy session is introduced to help manage patients' symptoms, this should be considered when evaluating the risks of the overall programme. Any supplementary interventions with potential clinical benefits for patients should also be targeted at groups who would benefit most, especially when they cannot be provided to all patients. For example, the one-time respiratory therapy session might be focused on patients who suffer from chronic pulmonary problems (provided they are not excluded from the programme for being at increased risk).

Step five—*evaluate whether the interventions pose net risks to patients*—requires judging, again based on the available evidence, whether the risks of each individual intervention exceed the intervention's potential clinical benefits. If the answer to this question is yes, then the given intervention is said to pose "net risks" to the patient. One way of making this determination is to ask whether an "informed clinician" who is committed solely to the promoting the patients' best clinical interests would recommend that they undergo the intervention in question (Rid and Wendler 2011). If the clinician would recommend the intervention, it promotes the patients' clinical interests and thus does not pose net risks. This implies that the intervention's risk-benefit profile is acceptable and—assuming the requirements of the previous steps are satisfied—needs no further evaluation. If the clinician would be indifferent, then undergoing the intervention neither undermines nor promotes the patients' clinical interests. Provided that including the intervention in the rational use programme is necessary to ensure its safety (step 2), this suggests that it has an acceptable risk-benefit profile. If the clinician would advise against the intervention, then it poses net risks that require further evaluation (step 6). For example, an informed clinician who is committed solely to promoting the patients' best clinical interests would not recommend delaying or withholding antibiotics for LRTIs (at least where the expected benefit of antibiotic treatment outweighs the expected harms of adverse effects of antibiotics outlined above). This means that this intervention poses net risks whose acceptability needs to be considered further.

Finally, step six—*evaluate whether the net risks to patients are justified by the programme's social value*—serves precisely this purpose. It first requires determining the cumulative level of net risk of the given rational use programme by adding the net risks of all its interventions. For example, restricting antibiotics for LRTIs likely poses a relatively small level of cumulative net risk from delaying or withholding antibiotic treatment and providing patients with written information in order to manage the resulting risks. Evaluators must then judge whether the programme's cumulative net risks fall within the general range of acceptable net risk to patients and, if the answer is yes, whether the risks are proportionate to the social value of implementing the programme.

With regard to the general range of acceptable net risk, there is a long-standing debate about this issue in clinical research that can inform judgements about the acceptability of rational use programmes. Debate has been most intense in the context of research involving participants who cannot give their own informed consent, such as children or patients with dementia. Many ethical guidelines and regulations, as well as many research ethicists, endorse a "minimal risk" threshold for such research in order to protect participants from excessive net research risks (Emanuel et al. 2008; WMA 2013; CIOMS 2016). The precise interpretation of this threshold remains contested. However, a recent analysis of the existing literature identifies several "lessons learned" that are equally pertinent for the evaluation of rational use programmes (Rid 2014). Specifically, the most convincing definitions of minimal risk refer to the two basic components of research risk, likelihood and magnitude of research harm. Further, these definitions distinguish different magnitudes of harm (e.g. small, moderate, serious) and set approximate likelihood thresholds for each magnitude of harm, where the likelihood thresholds are anchored with numeric information (e.g. 1 per 100,000) derived from risk comparisons. For example, if the risks of participating in a charity soccer game are considered acceptable, and this activity is thought to be relevantly similar to clinical research, data on the risks of playing soccer can be used to anchor likelihood thresholds for different magnitudes of research harm. At present, comparator risks are best specified as the risks that average, healthy, normal individuals in different age groups face in riskier but still acceptable activities that are directed at benefiting others, such as playing soccer for charitable purposes in children. In practice, this implies that the most convincing definitions of the minimal risk threshold equate minimal net research risks with very low likelihoods of serious and moderate harm and modest likelihoods of small harm (Rid 2014). Using this threshold as a preliminary guide for evaluating the acceptability of rational use programmes, net risks such as those reported for delaying antibiotics for LRTIs would seem to qualify as minimal. Specifically, if the two main complications—empyema and pneumonia—are classified as moderate harms, the up to 10% likelihood that they will occur (Schuetz et al. 2009) is broadly consistent with the likelihood of moderate harms observed in appropriate comparator risks (Rid et al. 2010).

Similar arguments have been advanced in the debate about upper risk limits in research with competent consenting adults. Specifically, several authors suggest that these upper risk limits should be delineated in comparison to appropriate comparators risks for competent adults, such as emergency medical assistance (London 2006; Miller and Joffe 2009). In rational use programmes that require clinicians to obtain informed consent for delaying or withholding antibiotics, the range of acceptable net risks could be evaluated based on what levels of risk are considered acceptable in research involving competent consenting adults. However, all current rational use programmes that we are aware of proceed without the patients' informed consent (though individual doctors may discuss prescribing decisions with their patients and seek to understand patients' preferences), so that the minimal net risk threshold is more pertinent. Moreover, although some ethical guidelines allow a "minor increase" above minimal risk in research without consent when it is not possible to gather the necessary data in a less risky manner and the social and scientific value of the research is compelling (CIOMS 2016), the minor increase over minimal risk threshold remains underspecified in the research ethics literature. We therefore would not recommend applying it systematically in the context of rational use programmes.

With regard to judging whether the net risks of a given rational use programme are proportionate to the social value of implementing it, one way of making this judgment is to ask whether an "informed and impartial social arbiter" would recommend the programme in question after carefully considering the risks and potential benefits for all affected parties and giving everyone's claims fair consideration, while treating likc cases alike in similar areas of policy (Rid and Wendler 2011). This test provides no more than a heuristic to guide evaluators' judgment; however, the idea of a social arbiter helps to ensure that rational use programmes are evaluated just like other programmes or policies that impose some level of risk on individuals for the sake of realising an important social good—within clinical medicine, but also beyond. In the case of delaying or withholding antibiotics for LRTIs, the (arguably) minimal net risks that this programme involves for patients would seem proportionate to the importance of preserving antibiotic effectiveness and the potential of this programme to help curb AMR. Moreover, given that net risks are minimal, the programme could proceed without obtaining the patients' informed consent.

Potential Objections

Critics might argue that there are less invasive strategies for curbing the spread of AMR that we should exhaust before delaying or withholding antibiotics in clinical medicine, such as eliminating unnecessary antibiotic treatments, reducing antibiotic use in farming, and investing more, and more effectively, into research on new antibiotics. These other strategies should indeed be pursued with urgency, and there is little reason to believe that adopting rational use programmes would undermine them. However, given that AMR is now recognized as one of the major public health threats of the twenty-first century, it is essential to consider all approaches that could delay or prevent AMR in an ethically justifiable way. As this paper argues, rational use programmes that involve delaying or withholding antibiotics should become part of the conversation.

It might also be objected that few such programmes would satisfy the minimal risk threshold known from the context of clinical research. At this point, it is difficult to respond to this objection because few reliable data exist on patient outcomes when antibiotics are delayed or withdrawn. However, we have identified at least one case—restricting antibiotic use for LTRIs—where reasonable estimates suggest that the minimal risk threshold would be respected. As more data become available, more cases could follow. Moreover, our proposed ethical framework would also be helpful for evaluating rational use programmes that pose more than minimal risks to patients and therefore require obtaining their informed consent to participate. However, as mentioned, all current rational use programmes we are aware of proceed without obtaining the patients' informed consent, and we suspect this will stay the same in future. To be effective, rational use programmes need to be implemented as widely as possible—and in practice this is likely to be feasible only when patients are not asked to give their informed consent to having antibiotic treatment withheld or delayed. Given the considerable uncertainty about the social value of rational use programmes in terms of curbing AMR, and considering that such programmes are generally rolled out without requiring that clinicians obtain patients' informed consent, we would argue that rational use programmes should pose no more than limited net risks to patients until more evidence supports their social value.

Finally, some might argue that the present argument rests on an ethical framework for risk-benefit evaluations in clinical research that is not universally accepted. In particular, prominent research ethicists hold that clinician-investigators should generally not delay or withhold established effective treatments from patient-participants in clinical trials (Weijer and Miller 2004). This argument is based on the idea that clinician-investigators continue to have clinical obligations in the research context, which make it unacceptable for them to act against the best clinical interests of patient-participants by depriving them of proven effective interventions. And, it might be argued, if it is not acceptable to delay or withhold proven interventions in the research context, then it is not acceptable to do the same in rational use programmes. However, it is important to see that this latter position is not universally accepted in research ethics. This is because it cannot explain why it is justified for clinician-investigators to pose any net research risks to patient-participants—for example, by performing research-specific blood draws or biopsies that have no prospect of clinical benefit. After all, these interventions by definition do not promote the best clinical interests of patient-participants (Miller and Brody 2003). The ethical framework for risk-benefit evaluations that forms the basis of the present paper avoids this problem. It justifies why some level of carefully evaluated net risk can be imposed to patient-participants, namely because clinical research has important social value. Moreover, the framework applies the same standards for acceptable net risk to all research interventions, whether or not net risks result from delaying or withholding effective treatments or from performing research procedures without a prospect of clinical benefit (Rid and Wendler 2011). Thus, the ethical framework for risk-benefit evaluations in clinical research used here, while not universally accepted, is arguably more defensible than the existing alternatives.

Conclusion

For clinicians, rational use programmes can pose ethical conflicts when they involve delaying or withholding antibiotics and thereby compromise the clinical interests of their present patients for the sake of preserving antibiotic effectiveness for future patient populations. Such exceptions from the general norm that clinicians should always act in the best interests of the present patient need to be carefully developed and managed. In this paper, based on a comparison to clinical research, we presented an ethical framework that enables an explicit and transparent evaluation of the net risks that rational use programmes can pose to patients in order to address AMR. Because these evaluations require judgments about complex empirical facts and normative questions, it is essential that rational use programmes be developed transparently and with the involvement of patients, clinicians and other relevant stakeholders. This involvement would not only improve the quality of deliberations, but also help to ensure the fairness and legitimacy of the resulting policies and their successful implementation.

Finally, the rational use of antibiotics can only be one part of a comprehensive strategy to address the danger of AMR; other measures have to be pursued with equal urgency, including better infection control, comprehensive strategies to reduce antibiotics use in animals, and the development of new antibiotics.

Acknowledgments We thank Jonathan Grant, Harald Schmidt, David Wendler, James Wilson and Peter West-Oram, as well as the editors of this volume, Euzebiusz (Zeb) Jamrozik and Michael Selgelid, for comments on earlier versions of this manuscript. AB's and JL's work was supported by the Deutsche Forschungsgemeinschaft (grant BU 2450/2-1).

Disclaimer This work was completed as part of Annette Rid's official duties as an employee of the NIH Clinical Center. However, the opinions expressed are the authors's own. They do not represent any position or policy of the National Institutes of Health, Public Health Service, or Department of Health and Human Services.

Appendix: Ethical Framework for Rational Antibiotic Use

Clinical research			Restricted antibiotic use		
Step	Elements	Example	Step	Elements	Example
1. Ensure and enhance the study's social value	1. Ensure the study methods are sound	Study uses recognized scientific methods	***1. Ensure and enhance the policy's social value***	1. Ensure that restricting antibiotics use for the given condition is based on sound evidence and policy methods	Available data allow estimating the clinical and public health impact of restricting antibiotics use for lower respiratory tract infections Policy to restrict antibiotics use for lower respiratory tract infections is rigorously developed (e.g. policy analysis, stakeholder consultation) and judged to be feasible and effective
	2. Ensure the study passes a minimum threshold of social value	Study addresses a valuable question: liver cancer is a serious disease and few treatments exist		2. Ensure that restricting antibiotics use for the given condition passes a minimum threshold of social value	Restricted antibiotics use for lower respiratory tract infections has the potential to address antimicrobial resistance, a major public health problem
	3. Enhance the knowledge to be gained from the study	Could make specimens available for other research		3. Enhance the knowledge to be gained from the policy	Initiate research[a] to evaluate how restricted antibiotics use for lower respiratory tract infections affects prescription rates, clinical outcomes, antimicrobial resistance etc. and update policy as new evidence comes in Evaluate how the experience with restricting antibiotics use for lower respiratory tract infections can inform the management of antibiotic use for other conditions (e.g. urinary tract infection)

(continued)

Clinical research			Restricted antibiotic use		
Step	Elements	Example	Step	Elements	Example
2. Identify the research interventions	1. Determine which interventions address the study question(s) or protect subjects1)	Investigational drug, blood draws, CT scan, liver biopsy (with ultrasound)	***2. Identify the policy interventions***	1. Identify the policy intervention and any supplementary (non-routine) interventions to protect patients	Policy intervention: restricted antibiotics use for lower respiratory tract infections Supplementary interventions: provide relevant information to patients in writing (e.g. high fever and other signs of a worsening condition, steps to take in this situation), provide 1-time respiratory therapy session to manage symptoms Exclude routine clinical interventions from analysis: provide relevant information verbally, provide supportive measures for lower respiratory tract infections (e.g. mucolytics, inhalation, pain medication)
	2. Ensure research interventions are likely to yield important and non-duplicative information	Could consider whether a liver biopsy is important for answering the study question(s)		2. Ensure that each supplementary intervention is essential for protecting patients1)	Could consider whether written patient information is essential

3. Evaluate and reduce the risks to participants	1. Evaluate the risks of each research intervention	Liver biopsy poses a 8-35 per 100,000 risk of hematothorax	***3. Evaluate and reduce the risks to patients***	1. Evaluate the risks of the policy intervention and each supplementary intervention	Restricting antibiotics use for lower respiratory tract infections poses risks of i.e. increase of complications like pneumonia or empyema, which may require antibiotics and/or hospitalisation) Providing relevant information to patients in writing (rather than verbally) might cause mild anxiety
	2. Reasonably reduce the risks	Could consider whether liver biopsy is safer with 1-on-1 monitoring		2. Reasonably reduce the risks	Ensure that routine lower respiratory tract infections to treat condition are implemented (e.g. supportive measures) Ensure that serious harms, should they occur, are adequately managed at no financial cost to the patient (e.g. antibiotics and/or hospitalisation) and patients receive compensation for any lasting serious harms Actively monitor or exclude patient groups from policy who are at increased risk of complications or other serious harms (e.g. immunodeficieny) Instruct clinicians to exercise judgment in individual cases Reassure patients about written information sheet

(continued)

Clinical research			Restricted antibiotic use		
Step	Elements	Example	Step	Elements	Example
4. Evaluate and enhance the potential benefits for participants	1. Evaluate the potential clinical benefits of each research intervention	Only investigational drug: may reduce cancer	***4. Evaluate and enhance the potential benefits for patients***	1. Evaluate the potential clinical benefits of the policy intervention and each supplementary intervention	Restricting antibiotics use for lower respiratory tract infections spares patients the risks of treatment (e.g. diarrhea) 1-time respiratory therapy session helps to manage symptoms
	2. Enhance the potential clinical benefits	Could focus on advanced liver cancer patients		2. Enhance the potential clinical benefits	Could focus on patients with chronic pulmonary problems
5. Evaluate whether the interventions pose net risks	1. Determine whether the risks of each individual intervention exceed the intervention's potential clinical benefits (implies net risks): Would an *informed clinician* who is committed solely to promoting patients' clinical interests recommend the intervention?1)	*Informed clinician* would recommend investigational drug: no net risks *Informed clinician* would not recommend blood draws, CT scan, liver biopsy: net risks	***5. Evaluate whether the interventions pose net risks***	1. Determine whether the risks of each individual intervention exceed the intervention's potential clinical benefits (implies net risks): Would an *informed clinician* who is committed solely to promoting the patient's clinical interests recommend the intervention?	*Informed clinician* would not recommend withholding antibiotic treatment for lower respiratory tract infections and measures to manage the resulting risks (e.g. written information, active monitoring): net risks *Informed clinician* would recommend respiratory therapy session: no net risks
				2. Determine whether the unit of policy and supplementary interventions pose net risks: would an *informed clinician* recommend the unit of interventions?	*Informed clinician* would not recommend unit of interventions: potential clinical benefits of respiratory therapy session do not outweigh the risks of withholding antibiotic treatment and measures to manage the resulting risks
6. Evaluate whether the net risks are justified by the potential benefits of other interventions	1. Determine whether any of the interventions stand in a relation of strict scientific necessity or unity (unit of interventions)	Blood draws, CT scan, and investigational drug (presumed true for present purposes)	*N/A*	*Reason: The policy and supplementary interventions always stand in a relation of strict "policy necessity" (unit of interventions) because the supplementary interventions are considered essential for protecting patients' interests (step 2). The first element of this step is therefore unnecessary. The second element has been included in the previous step (step 5).*	
	2. Determine whether any units of interventions pose net risks: would an *informed clinician* recommend the unit(s) of interventions?	*Informed clinician* would recommend the above unit of interventions (stipulates that the potential clinical benefits of the investigational drug offset the drug's own risks and the risks of the blood draws and CT scan)			

7. Evaluate whether the remaining net risks are justified by the study's social value	1. Determine the level of cumulative net risk in the study: add any absolute, relative, indirect, and excess net risks	Considerable level of cumulative net risks from the liver biopsy	***6. Evaluate whether the net risks are justified by the policy's social value***	1. Determine the level of cumulative net risk posed to patients	Relatively small level of net risk from withholding antibiotic treatment and measures to manage the resulting risks
	2. Determine whether the study's cumulative net risks fall within the general range of acceptable net risk: could judge in light of net risk limits in biomedical research, notably the "minimal risk"[a] threshold in research without informed consent for rational use programmes that do not require clinicians to obtain the patient's informed consent and upper net risk limits in research for rational use programmes that require informed consent	Cumulative net risks probably fall within the general range of acceptable net risk for research with competent participants		2. Determine whether the policy's cumulative net risks fall within the general range of acceptable net risk: could judge in light of risk limits in biomedical research	Net risks from withholding antibiotic treatment for lower respiratory tract infections arguably falls within the range of acceptable net risk in clinical research and practice (i.e. the net risks arguably fall below the minimal risk threshold)
	3. Evaluate whether the given level of cumulative net risk is proportionate to the social value of conducting the study: would an *ideal social arbiter* recommend the study?	*Ideal social arbiter* would recommend the study (presumed true for present purposes)		3. Evaluate whether the given level of cumulative net risk is proportionate to the social value of implementing the policy: would an *ideal social arbiter* recommend the policy?	*Ideal social arbiter* may recommend the policy, given the importance of curbing antimicrobial resistance and the arguably minimal net risks to patients

The table shows how an existing framework for risk-benefit evaluations in clinical research (Rid and Wendler 2011) is adapted for the purposes of evaluating the risks of restricted antibiotic use. Example for clinical research: hypothetical phase 2 study of an investigational treatment for liver cancer, involving administration of the investigational drug, a series of blood draws, a CT scan, and a liver biopsy (taken without modifications from [Rid and Wendler 2011]). Example for restricted antibiotic use: hypothetical policy to restrict of antibiotic use for lower respiratory tract infections without obtaining the patients' informed consent

[a]Research to evaluate the impact of restricted antibiotics use for a given condition should be judged based on standard ethical criteria for research (CIOMS 2016; WMA 2013)

References

Adeyi, O. et al. 2017. Drug-resistant infections: A threat to our economic future (vol. 2): final report. Washington, DC. World Bank Group. http://documents.worldbank.org/curated/en/323311493396993758/final-report.

Andreasen, M. 2014. *Arbejdspapirer om antibiotikaresistens (Working papers on antibiotic resistance)*. Det Etiske Råd (Danish Ethics Council): Copenhagen.

Australian Department of Health. 2015. Responding to the threat of antimicrobial resistance: Australia's first national antimicrobial resistance strategy 2015–2019. Canberra.

Battin, M.P., L.P. Francis, J.A. Jacobson, et al. 2009. *The patient as victim and vector: Ethics and infectious disease*. New York: Oxford University Press.

Boucher, H.W., G.H. Talbot, D.K. Benjamin, et al. 2013. 10 × '20 Progress—Development of new drugs active against gram-negative bacilli: An update from the Infectious Diseases Society of America. *Clinical Infectious Diseases* 56: 1685–1694.

Bundesministerium für Gesundheit. 2011. Deutsche Antibiotikaresistenz-Strategie [German antibiotic resistance strategy]. Berlin.

Charani, E., R. Edwards, N. Sevdalis, et al. 2011. Behavior change strategies to influence antimicrobial prescribing in acute care: A systematic review. *Clinical Infectious Diseases* 53: 651–662.

Cohen, G., N. Daniels, and N. Eyal. 2015. *Identified versus statistical lives: An interdisciplinary perspective*. Oxford: Oxford University Press.

Costelloe, C., C. Metcalfe, A. Lovering, et al. 2010. Effect of antibiotic prescribing in primary care on antimicrobial resistance in individual patients: Systematic review and meta-analysis. *BMJ* 340: c2096.

Council for International Organizations of Medical Sciences, World Health Organization. 2016. International Ethical for Health-related Research Involving Humans. Geneva. https://cioms.ch/wp-content/uploads/2017/01/WEB-CIOMS-EthicalGuidelines.pdf. Accessed 26 Nov 2018.

Daneman, N., D.E. Low, A. McGeer, et al. 2008. At the threshold: Defining clinically meaningful resistance thresholds for antibiotic choice in community-acquired pneumonia. *Clinical Infectious Diseases* 46: 1131–1138.

Davey, P., E. Brown, E. Charani, et al. 2013. Interventions to improve antibiotic prescribing practices for hospital inpatients. *Cochrane Database of Systematic Reviews* 30 (4): CD003543.

Davies, S.C., J. Grant, and M. Catchpole. 2013. *The drugs don't work: A global threat*. London: Penguin.

Drive-AB. 2018. Driving reinvestment in research and development for antibiotics and responsible antibiotic use. http://drive-ab.eu. Accessed 26 Nov 2018.

Emanuel, E., C. Grady, R.A. Crouch, et al. 2008. *The Oxford textbook of clinical research ethics*. New York: Oxford University Press.

General Assembly of the United Nations. 2016. High-level meeting on antimicrobial-resistance. New York. http://www.un.org/pga/71/event-latest/high-level-meeting-on-antimicrobial-resistance/. Accessed 26 Nov 2018.

Kollef, M.H., and S.T. Micek. 2014. Rational use of antibiotics in the ICU: Balancing stewardship and clinical outcomes. *JAMA* 312: 1403–1404.

Little, P., M. Moore, J. Kelly, et al. 2014. Delayed antibiotic prescribing strategies for respiratory tract infections in primary care: Pragmatic, factorial, randomised controlled trial. *BMJ* 348: g1606.

Littmann, J., and B. Buyx. 2014. Antibiotikaresistenz. Ethische Aspekte einer drängenden Herausforderung. *Ethik in der Medizin* 27 (4): 301–314.

Littmann, J., and A. Buyx. 2018. Rationaler Antibiotikaeinsatz als ethische Herausforderung. *Bundesgesundheitsblatt*. https://doi.org/10.1007/s00103-018-2716-0.

Littmann, J., A. Buyx, and O. Cars. 2015. Antibiotic resistance: An ethical challenge. *International Journal of Antimicrobial Agents* 46 (4): 359–361.

Littmann, J., A. Rid, and A.M. Buyx. 2018. Tackling anti-microbial resistance: Ethical framework for rational antibiotic use. *European Journal of Public Health* 28 (2): 359–363.

London, A.J. 2006. Reasonable risks in clinical research: A critique and a proposal for the integrative approach. *Statistics in Medicine* 25 (17): 2869–2885.

Mandell, L., R. Wunderink, A. Anzueto, et al. 2007. Infectious Diseases Society of America/American Thoracic Society: Consensus guidelines on the Management of Community-Acquired Pneumonia in adults. *Clinical Infectious Diseases* 44: 27–72.

Metlay, J.P., G.W. Waterer, A.C. Long, et al. 2019. Diagnosis and treatment of adults with community-acquired pneumonia. An official clinical practice guideline of the American Thoracic Society and Infectious Diseases Society of America. *American Journal of Respiratory and Critical Care Medicine* 200 (7): e45–e67.

Millar, M. 2012. Constraining the use of antibiotics: Applying Scanlon's contractualism. *Journal of Medical Ethics* 38: 465–469.

Miller, F., and H. Brody. 2003. A critique of clinical equipoise. Therapeutic misconception in the ethics of clinical trials. *The Hastings Center Report* 33 (3): 19–28.

Miller, F.G., and S. Joffe. 2009. Limits to research risks. *Journal of Medical Ethics* 35: 445–449.

Oczkowski, S. 2017. Antimicrobial stewardship programmes: Bedside rationing by another name? *Journal of Medical Ethics* 43 (10): 1–4. https://doi.org/10.1136/medethics-2015-102785.

O'Neill, J. 2014. Review on antimicrobial resistance. Antimicrobial resistance: tackling a crisis for the health and wealth of nations. London.

Organisation for Economic Co-Operation and Development (OECD). 2018. Stemming the superbug tide: Just a few dollars more, OECD Health Policy Studies, OECD Publishing, Paris, https://doi.org/10.1787/9789264307599-en. Accessed 26 Nov 2018.

Outterson, K., J.H. Rex, T. Jinks, et al. 2016a. Accelerating global innovation to address antibacterial resistance: Introducing CARB-X. *Nature Reviews Drug Discovery* 15: 589.

Outterson, K., S.J. Hoffman, A. Ghafur, et al. 2016b. International cooperation to improve access to and sustain effectiveness of antimicrobials. *Lancet* 387: 296.

President's Council of Advisors on Science and Technology (PCAST). 2014. *Report to the President on combating antimicrobial resistance*. Washington: PCAST.

Public Health Agency of Canada. 2014. Antimicrobial resistance and use in Canada: a federal framework for action. Ottawa.

Rex, J.H. 2014. ND4BB: Addressing the antimicrobial resistance crisis. *Nature Reviews Microbiology* 12: 231–232.

Rid, A. 2014. Setting risk thresholds in research: Lessons from the debate about minimal risk. *Monash Bioethics Review* 32 (1–2): 63–85.

Rid, A., and D. Wendler. 2011. A framework for risk-benefit evaluations in biomedical research. *Kennedy Institute of Ethics Journal* 21 (2): 141–179.

Rid, A., E.J. Emanuel, and D. Wendler. 2010. Evaluating the risks of clinical research. *Journal of the American Medical Association* 304 (13): 1472–1479. https://doi.org/10.1001/jama.2010.1414.

Rid, A., J. Littmann, and A. Buyx. 2019. Evaluating the risks of public health programs: Rational antibiotic use and antimicrobial resistance. *Bioethics* 33 (7): 734–748.

Schuetz, P., M. Christ-Crain, R. Thomann, et al. 2009. Effect of procalcitonin-based guidelines vs standard guidelines on antibiotic use in lower respiratory tract infections: The prohosp randomized controlled trial. *JAMA* 302: 1059–1066.

Selgelid, M.J. 2007. Ethics and drug resistance. *Bioethics* 21: 218–229.

Spurling, G.K., C.B. Del Mar, and L. Dooley et al. 2013. Delayed antibiotics for respiratory infections. In: Cochrane database of systematic reviews, ed: Cochrane, 30(4): CD004417.

Sunstein, C. 1993. On analogical reasoning. *Harvard Law Review* 106: 741–791.

The White House. 2014. National strategy for combating antibiotic-resitant bacteria. Washington.

UK Department of Health. 2013. UK five year antimicrobial resistance strategy 2013 to 2018. London.

Weijer, C., and P. Miller. 2004. When are research risks reasonable in relation to anticipated benefits. *Nature Medicine* 10 (6): 570–573.

Wendler, D. 2010. Are physicians always obligated to act in the patient's best interests? *Journal of Medical Ethics* 36 (2): 66–70.

Wendler, D., and A. Rid. 2017. In defense of the social value requirement for clinical research. *Bioethics* 31 (2): 77–86.

Williams, J. 2015. World Medical Association: Medical ethics manual, 3rd Edition 2015. Ferney-Voltaire Cedex: World Medical Association. https://www.wma.net/wp-content/uploads/2016/11/Ethics_manual_3rd_Nov2015_en.pdf. Accessed 26 Nov 2018.

Wilson, M., and M. Tan. 2010. *Raising awareness for prudent use of antibiotics in animals: Position paper of the global alliance for the prudent use of antibiotics (APUA)*. Rome: APUA.

World Health Organization (WHO). 1985. *The rational use of drugs, report of the conference of experts*. Geneva: WHO Press.

———. 2011. *Global strategy for containment of antimicrobial resistance*. Geneva: WHO Press.

———. 2014. *Antimicrobial resistance – global report on surveillance*. Geneva: WHO Press.

———. 2015. *Worldwide country situation analysis: response to antimicrobial resistance*. Geneva: WHO Press.

World Medical Association (WMA). 2013. Declaration of Helsinki: Ethical principles for medical research involving human subjects. Helsinki. https://www.wma.net/policies-post/wma-declaration-of-helsinki-ethical-principles-for-medical-research-involving-human-subjects/. Accessed 26 Nov 2018.

7

Antibiotics and Animal Agriculture: The Need for Global Collective Action

Jonathan Anomaly

Keywords Drug Resistance · Political philosophy · Moral philosophy · Economics

The use of antibiotics in animal agriculture is steadily increasing, especially in developing countries. The European Union and a handful of developed countries have implemented policies to scale back the use of antibiotics, recognizing its role in the global rise of antibiotic resistance. But many farmers who raise animals live in poor countries without public health regulations, or work for large corporate entities that can move their operations to places with weak regulations. To minimize the careless use of antibiotics around the world, we need multi-lateral coordination between states on some common standards for the use of antibiotics in animals.

Introduction

Imagine a world in which every time you tied your shoes, you contributed to a process that resulted in the unintended suffering and death of thousands of people you'll never know.[1] In this world, like ours, shoelaces are useful: they save time, are a little cheaper than using Velcro ties, and more convenient than wearing slip-on shoes. But when everyone ties their shoes, lots of people die, and many more suffer.

This is a strange world to imagine, but it is a lot like the world we live in. The culprit isn't tying shoelaces, of course, but consuming factory farmed meat. Factory farms are wicked places – one of the last bastions of legally sanctioned cruelty toward animals. But more than this, they are bad for human health.

[1] Parts of the introduction are reprinted from an article that first appeared in *Compass*, the annual magazine of the Kenan Institute for Ethics at Duke University (2017).

J. Anomaly (✉)
University of Pennsylvania, Philadelphia, PA, USA
e-mail: anomaly@upenn.edu

Some antibiotics are given to cattle and pigs to marginally speed up their growth. The biological mechanisms through which antibiotics promote growth aren't well understood, but the use of antibiotics to promote growth does seem to work. More importantly, raising animals in densely packed conditions requires a steady dose of antibiotics to prevent infections that would otherwise run rampant.

Like many practices, there are benefits as well as costs: meat from factory farms is cheaper than meat from farms with free-range animals, often about half the price. This is partly because factory farms allow animals to occupy less space, which makes their production cheaper, and this savings is passed on to consumers.

Apart from its obvious benefits, factory farming produces many costs (Anomaly 2015). In this essay, I will focus on the threat that our use of antibiotics in animal agriculture poses for human health. Contrary to popular opinion, the problem is not that antibiotics are passed along from animals to people who eat them, and that this is bad for our health. Instead, the problem is that the more antibiotics we give to livestock, the more we encourage the emergence and spread of antibiotic-resistant bacteria in a microbial environment shared by animals and people (Marshall and Levy 2011; Spellberg et al. 2016).

Like all eukaryotic organisms, people pay a high price for sex: each child only shares half of her genes with each parent. But sexual reproduction seems to confer benefits by increasing variation in the immune system children inherit, thus making it more likely that some of them will survive the onslaught of parasites that continually evolve novel ways of exploiting their hosts (Hamilton et al. 1990). As strange as sex is – each of two independent organisms swapping their genes to create a hybrid – the bacterial equivalent is even kinkier than a San Francisco night club. Bacteria reproduce by cloning themselves, but they evolve throughout their lives by promiscuously swapping genes with other bacteria and by extracting genes from the viruses that parasitize them. This allows them to adapt to new environments quickly: in a lethal environment, a small number of bacteria are likely to have some advantage over the trillions that die. And this advantage comes either from a random genetic mutation, or from the lateral transfer of genes from one bacterium to another.

Some genes allow bacteria to fend off the antibiotics that plants, animals, and other bacteria use to destroy them. Many of these naturally occurring antibiotics have existed for billions of years, as part of an unending evolutionary arms race between host and parasite. Like their naturally occurring cousins, synthetic antibiotics made in a lab usually involve penetrating a bacterial cell wall and disrupting DNA synthesis, or otherwise slowing or stopping bacterial reproduction.

All a bacterium needs to survive an antibiotic is some way to either block the penetration of the chemical with a thick cell wall, degrade it with enzymes, or pump it out if it penetrates its body. Once that happens, it's off to the races. The lucky bacterium multiplies rapidly and spreads its resistance to other bacteria. When new resistant strains of bacteria emerge in animal agriculture, they are passed along to farmers who work with animals, workers who slaughter animals, consumers who eat meat, and people in our more general microbial environment (Laxminarayan et al. 2016).

The average person hosts about 40 trillion bacteria at any given time, and we constantly swap bacteria with each other and with the environment around us (Sender et al. 2016). So even though the overuse of antibiotics tends to affect those closest to the source of resistant bacteria – whether animals or people – over time, strains of bacteria that are resistant to antibiotics can spread through trade and travel among people, and through soil and streams around factory farms. And while reducing the use of antibiotics does tend to reduce resistance, the decline of resistance does not happen immediately, since reservoirs of antibiotic-resistant genes tend to persist in bacterial plasmids for a long time (Andersson and Hughes 2010).

For more than a decade the European Union has banned antibiotics for growth promotion in farm animals, and tried to impose standards that increase animal welfare and reduce the need to use antibiotics. The US has begun to follow suit, driven by consumer demand for antibiotic-free meat, and FDA threats of regulation. But most developing countries are moving in the opposite direction, with explosive growth of antibiotic use in both people and animals in China, India, Pakistan, Egypt, and many sub-Saharan African countries (Van Boeckel et al. 2015).

Economic Models

The problem of antibiotic resistance is often framed by well-known economic models like the prisoner's dilemma, the tragedy of the commons, or the provision of public goods. All three models are useful in some contexts, but when they are not adequately qualified they can cast shade rather than light on the problem of resistance.

Prisoner's Dilemma

Consider first the prisoner's dilemma (PD). In the original example, we are presented with two prisoners who are suspected of armed robbery, but a District Attorney (DA) who only has enough evidence to prosecute them for the illegal possession of firearms. The prisoners are in separate jail cells, and the DA offers each of them a deal: if you snitch on your accomplice and he stays silent, you'll get off scot free and he'll be executed. If you both stay silent, you'll each get one year in prison. If you both snitch, you'll each get a decade in prison. The payoffs are as follows:

Odin	Loki	
	Silence	Snitch
Silence	1 year/1 year	Death/Freedom
Snitch	Freedom/Death	10 years/10 years

If the accomplices lack friendly feelings for one another, and if neither fears reprisals outside of prison, the rational move for each is to snitch, even if the socially optimal move is for both to stay silent. The PD is interesting because each player acting rationally produces an outcome that is worse for everyone.

The PD is a simple model that is frequently invoked to explain why rational agents act in ways that contribute to air pollution or species extinction even when each person would prefer to breath clean air or preserve biodiversity. Although most of the real-world games the PD is used to illustrate are complicated by the fact that there are more than two players, that players have asymmetric information or poorly formed preferences, and that they face uncertainty about whether (or how many times) the game will be repeated, the simplistic two player model is still of some use in visualizing problems like antibiotic resistance.

Consider the following case. Each carnivore faces the choice to consume meat from factory farmed animals or humanely raised animals free from antibiotics.

Odin	Loki	
	Humanely raised	Factory farmed
Humanely raised	2nd/2nd	4th/1st
Factory farmed	1st/4th	3rd/3rd

The payoff matrix indicates that each person does best by consuming factory farmed meat, that each does worst by consuming humanely raised meat (if the other does not), but that they both do better if they both consume meat from humanely raised rather than factory farmed animals. In the real world, if there were only two consumers and two producers, the effects of Loki's consumption choices would not be big enough to adversely affect Odin's welfare. But when we generalize to hundreds of millions of people, we get a case in which each person marginally increases the probability of antibiotic-resistant bacteria emerging and spreading, but each also saves a bit of money by consuming meat from factory farmed animals. As long as the benefit to each from buying factory farmed meat exceeds the costs associated with the alternative, the model predicts they will continue their socially suboptimal behavior.

There are several limitations of extending a two-person model to a many-person case. First, in the large number case we can treat other people's actions as given, whereas in the small number case we might change their behavior by reasoning with them (Bowles and Gintis 2013). Second, in the large number case we may have to resort to using state power to incentivize socially optimal behavior, whereas in the small number case people are in a better position to create local solutions that exploit social norms and informal punishments to move from the Nash equilibrium to the Pareto optimum (Ostrom 2000).

Similar considerations apply to farmers choosing whether to raise their animals with or without antibiotics, which is a many-person prisoner's dilemma in which most people reason parametrically (taking other's actions as more-or-less given). While there is a growing market for antibiotic-free meat, so that some farmers find it profitable to reject factory farming, most consumers around the world either don't know enough or care enough about the problem to entice farmers to reject antibiotics and raise their animals humanely.

Tragedy of the Commons

Many have argued that our aggregate use of antibiotics – in hospital settings and animal agriculture – is analogous to the misuse of commonly owned resources. In the classic example of a commons tragedy, farmers lack private property rights and are forced to raise animals on a common plot of land. The farmers internalize the benefits from raising animals and selling their meat, but share the costs of grass and soil depletion. Consequently, in the absence of sufficient altruistic restraint, each farmer continues to add animals to the commons up to the point at which the personal benefits equal the personal costs. To the extent that they ignore social costs, farmers add animals even if it makes everyone worse off than they would be if they agreed to a set of enforceable constraints.

Assume, for example, that above some number for each animal added to a common pasture, each farmer will get 10 utility points but the community will lose 20 utility points as the grass becomes overgrazed. If there are 10 farmers, each nets 8 utility points from adding another animal (+10 from selling the meat and – 2 from depleting grass and soil), and so they add animals until the commons is ruined. The typical solution to commons tragedies is to privatize plots of land, or (less efficiently) to set up enforceable limits with penalties for exceeding the limits. In small settings, these standards can be enforced by the court of public opinion, assuming farmers care about their reputation in the community. In large settings, standards are usually set by the state, and enforced with penalties for violating laws, or taxes and subsidies that attempt to bring about a socially optimal use of common resources.

Is the use of antibiotics on factory farms a commons tragedy? Some suggest that it is (Hollis and Maybarduk 2015). Others are more cautious, arguing that it depends on assumptions that include how quickly alternative antibiotics and vaccines will be developed, and how accurately we can diagnose infections (McAdams 2017a). Just as there is no such thing as a precise carrying capacity for land (since we can develop chemical fertilizers to increase soil productivity, or genetically engineer animals to more efficiently turn grass into meat), so too there is no specific point at which using more antibiotics necessarily imposes net costs on people.

As with the Prisoner's Dilemma, the commons tragedy model can help us conceptualize the incentives that generate the problem of antibiotic resistance. But it can also be misleading. For example, suppose we develop better diagnostics. Rapid diagnostic tests can make broad-spectrum antibiotics last longer by helping us identify the specific kind of infection plaguing a person or animal so that we can treat it with a narrow-spectrum antibiotic agent (McAdams 2017a). When better diagnostics are available to guide treatment in conjunction with extremely narrow-spectrum agents, David McAdams argues that "greater antibiotic use can in some cases decrease the selective pressure favoring resistant bacteria" (2017a, p. 6). Better diagnostics may also make it more profitable for companies to manufacture and conserve antibiotics if it leads physicians and farmers to more carefully use antibiotics to target specific infections (2017b). Using the wrong antibiotic often fails to treat the relevant infection, and it encourages resistance among all bacteria that the antibiotic affects. Using broad-spectrum antibiotics without a specific diagnosis is like carpet-bombing an entire city in order to kill a few soldiers. To the extent that we can target our enemies with precision strikes, there is less opportunity for collateral damage in the form of resistant strains of bacteria that grow in number as their susceptible compatriots are killed.

In addition to rapid diagnostic tests, the invention of "adjuvants" (supplements that make antibiotics more effective by priming our immune system, or by blocking bacterial resistance) can extend the life of antibiotics (Wright 2016). Rapid diagnostics and effective adjuvants show that the collective consumption of antibiotics does not *automatically* create a commons tragedy. It all depends on how we use antibiotics, and this is in part a function of technology, and the incentives that physicians and farmers face as a result of public policies.

Nevertheless, the careless way in which antibiotics are currently used in animal agriculture outside of Europe probably *is* a commons tragedy. This is because farmers in most countries today simply ignore the social cost of using antibiotics in livestock, and many farmers fail to understand how using antibiotics in agriculture can lead to the rise of bacterial infections in people that are increasingly expensive, difficult, or impossible to treat.

Public Goods

A final model frequently used to describe problems associated with our use of antibiotics requires us to make a distinction. In economics, *private* goods are those that are consumed by individuals in ways that don't involve significant externalities (costs or benefits borne by people external to an economic transaction). For example, when I buy a private good like a cup of coffee or a pair of eyeglasses, the costs or benefits imposed on other people are trivial. *Public* goods, by contrast, are consumed in common, so that we share the benefits of consumption. Public goods can be thought of as non-excludable positive externalities (Cowen 2008), though this is misleading in cases where the public good is experienced as a cost rather than a benefit to those who consume it.

Antibiotics themselves are not public goods, but to some extent the *efficacy* of antibiotics, and efforts made to move us toward the socially optimal use of antibiotics, *are* public goods. Similarly, efforts to eliminate infectious diseases are public goods (Selgelid 2007), since the reduction or eradication of a disease is shared by all people in a region, and potentially all people on the planet. By extension, reducing the reckless use of antibiotics in agriculture is a public good. Although alternative agricultural methods are more expensive, the enormous external costs of drug-resistant diseases that emerge from factory farming almost certainly exceed the benefits of cheaper meat (O'Neill et al. 2015).[2]

Many people, including some economists, equate public goods problems with commons tragedies and prisoner's dilemmas. This is a mistake, although it is understandable since many commons tragedies and public goods problems can be usefully modeled by the prisoner's dilemma. But often public goods are better described as assurance games or coordination games (Hampton 1987), and this is good news for lawmakers and farming associations who are aware of the problem and want to converge on common standards that allow them to make a profit *and* minimize the risk of antibiotic resistance. One problem with preserving global public goods like the efficacy of antibiotics is that most people are unaware of the problem, since each plays a very small role in producing it. In other words, many people who might help preserve or produce public goods are rationally ignorant about the nature of the problem.

Moral Principles

Ignorance of how the use of antibiotics in agriculture harms human health is *rational* in the economic sense, but it is not necessarily *morally excusable* (Anomaly 2015). Since the problem of AMR is difficult to understand, and since each act of consuming factory-farmed products contributes only imperceptibly to the problem, it makes perfect sense that consumers would ignore the problem and purchase cheap factory-farmed meat, rather than more expensive meat from farms that don't use antibiotics.

But the fact that we can explain consumer ignorance does not absolve consumers of responsibility for contributing to the problem. As information about the private benefits and social costs of using antibiotics in farm animals becomes more widely available, consumers have an increasing responsibility to act on it by changing their purchasing habits and trying to persuade governments to make it harder to purchase meat from animals unnecessarily dosed with antibiotics. Alexander Fleming

[2] It may be that *some* use of antibiotics in agriculture is both individually beneficial for animals (who contract infections despite humane and prudent farming practices), and socially beneficial for people (who may be less likely to contract a bacterial infection an animal has). But the growing quantity of antibiotics used in farming today is likely to produce harms that far exceed these benefits.

famously warned that "the thoughtless person playing with penicillin is morally responsible for the death of the man who finally succumbs to infection with the penicillin-resistant organism."[3] One form of "playing with penicillin" is the use of it as a growth promoter on factory farms, or the more common use of it to prevent infections in the cramped and cruel conditions that characterize factory farms.

A more nuanced version of Fleming's admonition requires us to distinguish *actual* harms to discrete people from *probabilistic* harms to actual or potential people. Another way to put the point is to say that the harms of antibiotic resistance are "identity-independent" in the sense that the victims of AMR cannot be known ahead of time and, in some cases, are not yet born. While a single farmer (or consumer) misusing antibiotics can create or encourage a resistant strain that spreads to other people, generally the prevalence of resistant bacteria in the environment depends on how all of us act. By acting in ways that create genetic pollution in our microbial environment, we make it a little more likely that someone will suffer or die of a previously treatable infection.

Many other pollution problems are structurally similar to antibiotic resistance. For example, each of us drives to work and produces the social costs of pollution and traffic congestion as a byproduct, while experiencing the private benefit of an enjoyable ride in our own car. There are also *social* benefits when each person drives, if driving contributes to a more efficient workforce that creates better goods at lower cost. Suppose the social costs of air pollution and traffic congestion exceed the individual benefits of driving. A common response is to impose a price on driving by taxing fuel or charging user fees to encourage the efficient use of roads and the atmosphere. The underlying moral principles are that we should pay in proportion to the amount we contribute to the problem, and that if anyone's liberties to pollute are restricted, then all us should face the same restrictions (Gaus 1999, p. 197).

Similar arguments have been made for taxing antibiotics in medicine and agriculture to discourage low-value use (Kades 2005; Anomaly 2013). But antibiotic resistance is much more complicated than air pollution or traffic congestion: in some cases we may want to *subsidize* rather than *tax* the use of antibiotics when people who can't afford them are likely to spread infectious diseases to others (Selgelid 2007). Apart from taxes and subsidies, there is a vast literature on how to harness intellectual property rights, prescription requirements, basic science research funding, and shared surveillance to control the problem (O'Neill et al. 2016).

What I now want to argue is that without more coordination between states, the problem of antibiotic resistance in agriculture will likely get worse, with dire consequences for human health in the coming century.

---

[3] http://www.fda.gov/NewsEvents/Speeches/ucm427312.htm

Global Coordination

The provision of global public goods like conserving antibiotics and reducing infectious disease raises two problems: the *free rider* problem occurs when individual consumers, farmers, or states seek the gains of limited antibiotic use without paying the costs; the *assurance* problem occurs when each is willing to pay the cost of reducing unnecessary use, but lacks the assurance that others will abide by policies that constrain our collective use of antibiotics.

The first problem is difficult to overcome to the extent that self-interest dominates the actions of farmers in a market or of politicians in a government. But there is some evidence that most consumers who understand the problem are willing to pay higher prices for meat from animals not given antibiotics (Spellberg et al. 2016). Moreover, if people really understood the problems factory farms create they would likely be willing to pay significantly more for meat, since most people support taxes (or costly regulations) when they are reasonably sure the tax will be used to discourage the problems associated with pollution (Kallbekken et al. 2011).

Agricultural producers are also likely to be willing to comply with standards that limit antibiotic use provided other firms are also forced to internalize the cost of similar regulations or taxes. The fact that the assurance problem is often more serious than the free rider problem in trying to elicit cooperation in many public goods games (Bowles and Gintis 2013) is good news for those who worry about the feasibility of states setting mutually beneficial standards.

Part of the problem with antibiotics in agriculture is that as transportation costs decline, the market for animal meat becomes increasingly global: animal feed is produced in one country, animals are raised in another, and then meat is exported to a third country. Since producers in many countries are now in a position to operate industrial animal farms, unless all states set standards that limit antibiotic use, producers will tend to migrate to countries with the weakest regulations. There is already some evidence that this "race to the bottom" is happening as Chinese farms are producing meat in factory farms that use more confinement and antibiotics than farms in other countries. In fact, just as the US is beginning to move away from factory farming due to consumer demand and threats of regulation by the US Food and Drug Administration, many of the most populous developing countries – including China, India, and Brazil – are embracing factory farming (O'Neill et al. 2015).

A well-designed trade treaty between major exporters and importers of meat should recognize the problem of "leakage," which occurs when one country sets relatively high environmental standards, and allows other countries with weaker standards to increase the production of similar goods in ways that simply changes where the pollution is emitted (Barrett 1999). In other words, any treaty worth implementing cannot reward free-riding countries whose firms are permitted to externalize the costs of their production, while firms in other countries internalize the costs of complying with policies that would make everyone better off if countries complied with them.

A second feature of an effective treaty to limit antibiotics in agriculture is a minimum participation clause to assure prospective signatories that unless a sufficient number of nations sign on, they will not be forced to pay additional production costs (Barrett 1999). This feature solves the assurance problem for firms and nations that are willing to comply with stricter production practices provided enough others do to produce the global benefits associated with restricting antibiotic use.

A third feature of any multi-lateral agreement to restrict antibiotic use is that it would need to be flexible enough to allow countries to achieve collective goals in different ways. For example, some experts advocate setting targets for the *per capita* quantity of antibiotics that can be administered to animals. According to the British Review on Antimicrobial Resistance, pork producers in Denmark (the first country to ban antibiotics as growth promoters) use about 50 mg of antibiotics per kg of livestock in the country (O'Neill et al. 2015, p. 2).

A flexible treaty would take something like this number as a benchmark that all countries must meet, but it would allow countries to achieve the relevant goal in different ways: by taxing antibiotics, placing a cap on total use, restricting antibiotics by requiring veterinary oversight, or some combination of these policies. Antibiotics deemed especially important for human use should probably be banned for use in agriculture by all countries. But what often matters is the *quantity* of antibiotics used, not just the *kind*. This is especially true because plasmids that confer antibiotic resistance can be transferred between bacteria of different species, and can reduce the efficacy of different drugs than those administered by farmers (Marshall and Levy 2011).

One advantage of imposing "pollution taxes" or user fees on antibiotics in agriculture is that, unlike regulations, governments have strong incentives to enforce them. Governments can use the revenue raised from taxes to finance vaccination programs that minimize the need to administer antibiotics. They might also fund basic science research that aims to develop new vaccines and diagnostics for infectious diseases, and to develop entirely new treatments like genetically engineered bacteriophage viruses (Bikard et al. 2014).

Taxing socially costly activities like using antibiotics in agriculture also incentivizes farmers to find alternative ways to produce meat that minimize antibiotic resistance. These alternatives may include increasing the roaming space animals have, and decreasing the stress they face when forced to live in extreme confinement. A more promising alternative is to create "in vitro meat" made in a lab from embryonic stem cells. This would avoid the need to raise animals at all, thus reducing untold amounts of suffering and potential public health problems.

Finally, any agreement to restrict antibiotic use should be attractive enough for each participating country to be willing to *enforce* it. It is likely that offering benefits for compliance will be more effective than simply threats of sanctions for noncompliance. For example, it is in the interest of all nations that each nation monitors the outbreak and spread of infectious diseases, as well as novel patterns of antibiotic resistance. But sometimes only wealthier states have the budgets and technology to accomplish this. By sharing information and technology with developing countries, wealthier countries can both signal goodwill and deliver tangible benefits to other countries they wish to comply with stricter controls on antibiotic use. This may act as a positive incentive for poor countries to do their part, even if the threat of sanctions for non-compliance with collectively beneficial restrictions is also important.

Each nation faces its own challenges, including an electorate that is unlikely to fully understand the social benefits and costs of antibiotics, and factory farmers who are unlikely to welcome regulations that impose new costs on them. Governments can justify spending some money to ease the transition from factory farming techniques to alternatives that produce better consequences for the same reason they can justify compensating taxi cab drivers who were required to buy a costly permit from the state to drive a taxi, but who are now forced to compete with companies like Uber, whose drivers did not have to pay for the right to operate as a taxi service. In fact, if relatively wealthy governments offer temporary assistance to domestic firms to transition away from factory farming, and to relatively poor governments to comply with new restrictions, the move away from the reckless use of antibiotics may be easier to induce, and more fair from the standpoint of global distributive justice.

References

Andersson, Dan, and Diarmaid Hughes. 2010. Antibiotic resistance and its cost: Is it possible to reverse resistance? *Nature* 8: 260–271.

Anomaly, Jonathan. 2013. Collective action and individual choice. *Journal of Medical Ethics* 39: 752–756.

———. 2015. What's wrong with factory farming? *Public Health Ethics* 8 (3): 246–254.

Barrett, Scott. 1999. Montreal vs Kyoto. In *Global public goods: International cooperation for the 21st century*, ed. Inge Kaul et al. Oxford: Oxford University Press.

Bikard, David, et al. 2014. Exploiting CRISPR-Cas nucleases to produce sequence-specific antimicrobials. *Nature Biotechnology* 32: 1146–1150.

Bowles, Samuel, and Herbert Gintis. 2013. *A cooperative species: Human reciprocity and its evolution*. Princeton: Princeton University Press.

Cowen, Tyler. 2008. *Public goods. The concise encyclopedia of economics*. 2nd ed. http://www.econlib.org/library/Enc/PublicGoods.html.

Gaus, Gerald. 1999. *Social philosophy*. London: M.E. Sharpe Publishing.

Hamilton, William, et al. 1990. Sexual reproduction as an adaptation to resist parasites. *Proceedings of the National Academy of Science* 87: 3566–3573.

Hampton, Jean. 1987. Free rider problems in the production of collective goods. *Economics and Philosophy* 3: 245–273.

Hollis, Aidan, and Peter Maybarduk. 2015. Antibiotic resistance is a tragedy of the commons that necessitates global cooperation. *Journal of Law, Medicine, and Ethics* 43: 33–37.

Kades, Eric. 2005. Preserving a precious resource: Rationalizing the use of antibiotics. *Northwest University Law Review* 99: 611–675.

Kallbekken, Steffen, et al. 2011. Do you not like Pigou, or do you not understand him? *Journal of Environmental Economics and Management* 62 (1): 53–64.

Laxminarayan, Ramanan, et al. 2016. Antibiotic use and resistance in food animals. *The Center for Disease Dynamics, Economics, and Policy*. https://cddep.org/sites/default/files/india_abx_report.pdf. Accessed 1 May 2017.

Marshall, Bonnie, and Stuart Levy. 2011. Food animals and antimicrobials: Impacts on human health. *Clinical Microbiology Reviews* 24 (4): 718–733.

McAdams, David. 2017a. Resistance diagnosis and the changing epidemiology of antibiotic resistance. *New York Academy of Sciences.* 1388 (2017): 5–17.

———. 2017b. Resistance diagnosis and the changing economics of antibiotic discovery. *New York Academy of Sciences.* 1388 (2017): 18–25.

O'Neill, Jim, et al. 2015. Antimicrobials in agriculture and the environment: Reducing unnecessary use and waste. *The Review on Antimicrobial Resistance*. http://amr-review.org/.

———. 2016. Tackling drug-resistant infections globally: Final report and recommendations. *The Review on Antimicrobial Resistance*. http://amr-review.org/.

Ostrom, Elinor. 2000. Collective action and the evolution of social norms. *Journal of Economic Perspectives* 14 (3): 137–158.

Selgelid, Michael. 2007. Ethics and drug resistance. *Bioethics* 21 (4): 218–229.

Sender, Ron, et al. 2016, August 19. Revised estimates for the number of human and bacterial cells in the body. *PLOS Biology*. https://doi.org/10.1371/journal.pbio.1002533.

Spellberg, Brad, et al. 2016. *Antibiotic resistance in humans and animals*. Discussion paper for the National Academy of Medicine. Accessed May 2017. http://www.nam.edu/antibiotic-resistance-in-humans-and-animals.

Van Boeckel, T.P., et al. 2015. Global trends in antimicrobial use in food animals. *Proceedings of the National Academy of Sciences* 112 (18): 5649–5654.

Wright, Gerard. 2016. Antibiotic adjuvants: Rescuing antibiotics from resistance. *Trends in Microbiology* 24 (11): 862–871.

8

Fairness in the Use of Information About Carriers of Resistant Infections

John G. Francis and Leslie P. Francis

Abstract One standard menu of approaches to the prevalence of anti-microbial resistance diseases is to enhance surveillance, fund research to develop new antimicrobials, and educate providers and patients to reduce unnecessary antimicrobial use. The primarily utilitarian reasoning behind this menu is unstable, however, if it fails to take fairness into account. This chapter develops an account of the fair uses of information gained in public health surveillance. We begin by sketching information needs and gaps in surveillance. We then demonstrate how analysis of information uses is incomplete if viewed from the perspectives of likely vectors of disease who may be subjects of fear and stigma and likely victims who may be coerced into isolation or quarantine. Next, we consider aspects of fairness in the use of information in non-ideal circumstances: inclusive participation in decisions about information use, resource plans for those needing services, and assurances of reciprocal support. Fairness in information use recognizes the ineluctable twinning of victims and vectors in the face of serious pandemic disease.

Keywords Fairness · Data use · Privacy · Surveillance

As many chapters in this volume emphasize, the prevalence of anti-microbial resistant diseases and the comparative paucity of available treatments presents a public health crisis. One standard menu of approaches to this crisis is to enhance surveillance to gain information needed to identify potential disease vectors and to ascertain likely modes of transmission; to fund research to develop new treatments and

J. G. Francis
Department of Political Science, University of Utah, Salt Lake City, USA
e-mail: john.francis@utah.edu

L. P. Francis (✉)
College of Law & Department of Philosophy, University of Utah, Salt Lake City, USA
e-mail: francisl@law.utah.edu

antimicrobials; and to intervene through education, treatment, and careful stewardship of the existing antimicrobials that retain some efficacy. This combination of approaches is founded primarily in utilitarian reasoning, attempting to achieve the best possible mitigation of the current crisis in the hopes that effective new treatment methods may soon become available.

Such utilitarian reasoning is not entirely stable in practice, however. On the one hand, when the prospects of exposure to untreatable and potentially fatal disease appear imminent, fear may become the overriding reaction to those who are identified as ill. The result may be forms of coercion against people suspected of being vectors of disease that appear prudential in the short term but that are insufficiently grounded in science and potentially counter-productive in the longer term. People may hide to avoid disclosure and deleterious consequences of over-regulation may lead to under-regulation. Recent examples include demands to compel isolation of people believed to have been exposed to Ebola or for banning travel from regions where outbreaks of conditions such as Ebola or Zika have been identified. On the other hand, concerns for victims may generate outpourings of resources for treatment, calls for investment in public health resources in underserved areas, and renewed emphasis on privacy protections. These too may be counterproductive if they result in confusion and waste of resources or multiple conflicting strategies. The upshot may be policies that oscillate between treating people as vectors and treating them as victims but without significant or coordinated progress against the problem of resistance.

Each of these perspectives—victim-hood and vector-hood—is morally important. But in our judgment analysis that is limited to these perspectives is incomplete in its failure to take certain considerations of fairness into account. Our specific focus here is the use of information, but similar points could be made about other types of resources as well. Collection, uses, and access to information, we contend in what follows, must be rooted in the effort to make progress against serious public health problems in a manner that is reasonably fair under the circumstances. This requires not only concern for people as victims and vectors but concerns about how the impact of policies are distributed and foster cooperative connections in both the shorter and the longer term.

The Important Roles of Information

Traditional public health surveillance methods are both individual and population based. Where particular individuals are concerned, the role of information is primarily to enable strategies to interrupt disease transmission. Case identification, case reporting, contact tracing, treatment if possible, and education and intervention if needed to prevent transmission come to the fore. At every stage, information is critical. If individuals with transmissible disease are unknown or cannot be located, efforts to interrupt transmission will fail. Efforts will also fail if information is not transmitted to those who are capable of acting, whether they be authorities designated to enforce quarantine or isolation or health care personnel equipped to offer treatment or prophylaxis. Education requires information, too, about where to direct educational efforts and what these efforts might contain. Importantly, if people who might suffer exposures are insufficiently informed about the likelihood and seriousness of contagion and the need for precautions, they may unwittingly become infected vectors as well as victims themselves. Such was the case for health care workers during the SARS epidemic of 2003 and for many during the Ebola epidemic of 2014.

Information gleaned in population-level surveillance plays many additional important roles in addressing the problem of anti-microbial resistance. A longstanding recommendation of the WHO, codified in the World Health Regulations that entered into force in 2007 in article 44, is international cooperation in the development of surveillance capacities for the identification of potential global health emergencies of international concern (WHO 2005). Surveillance can help to identify rates of incidence and prevalence of resistant disease. Testing samples can yield information about histories and patterns of disease spread. Samples also can be used to identify biological characteristics of resistant infectious agents that may be helpful in developing methods of treatment or identifying new anti-microbial agents.

Population level surveillance can be targeted to identifying the incidence and prevalence of resistant disease in particular geographical areas. Gonorrhea is an example. There were 78.3 million estimated new cases of gonorrhea worldwide in 2012; the highest number occurred in low-income areas of the western Pacific. Resistant disease has become increasingly prevalent, especially in these areas and among groups such as sex workers and truck drivers (Unemo et al. 2017). Extensively drug-resistant (XDR) gonorrhea cases also have appeared in Spain and in France, although these strains do not appear to have spread, possibly because they are less hardy and so less likely to be passed on. However, significant resistance may not be detected because of "suboptimal antimicrobial resistance surveillance in many settings" (Unemo et al. 2017). A recent international panel reviewing resistant gonorrhea recommends strategies of case management, partner notification, screening (especially of sex workers and men having sex with men), and evidence-based treatment (Unemo et al. 2017); these recommendations are based on surveillance data.

Population-level surveillance information may also be useful in identifying risks associated with providing humanitarian treatment. Over 30,000 young people wounded in the Libyan civil war that began in 2011 were evacuated elsewhere for treatment. Concerns arose that many of these patients were recognized to carry with them resistant organisms—thus bringing along with their needs for treatment risks to other patients being treated in the host facilities (Zorgani and Ziglam 2013). Institutions accepting these patients were informed of this risk so that they could take appropriate precautions. Libya itself was identified as a region with high prevalence of resistant organisms, despite the limited surveillance capacities in that conflict-torn nation. Recommendations included improving surveillance in Libya—which lacks a national surveillance system—and implementation of infection prevention measures in Libyan hospitals.

Surveillance is also used to identify practices that might contribute to the development of resistance. Use of antimicrobials in agriculture is one area of inquiry, although its precise contribution to the problem is not easy to quantify (e.g. Hoelzer et al. 2017). There have been many studies of problematic prescribing practices among physicians in the US (Wigton et al. 2008), Europe (e.g. Jørgensen et al. 2013), Asia (Lam and Lam 2003), and elsewhere (Trap and Hansen 2002), along with efforts to educate physicians about appropriate antimicrobial use.

Ever since the recognition grew that crowds celebrating the return of soldiers from World War I had created a ready opportunity for transmission of the Spanish influenza, epidemiologists have observed the potential health risks of large gatherings that concentrate people together, even for brief periods of time. Examples include music festivals, major sporting competitions, other large festivals, and religious gatherings such as the Hajj or other pilgrimages. The largest estimated gathering is the periodic Kumbh Mela pilgrimage in which Hindus come together to bathe in a sacred river such as the Ganges; over 40 million people, drawn largely from the Indian subcontinent but increasingly international, attend the event (Gautret and Steffen 2016). The largest annual gathering of pilgrims is the Hajj at Mecca which draws over two million people; the Fifth Pillar of Islam is the obligation to undertake the once in a lifetime journey for those who can physically or financially afford to do so. With such great numbers of people together for sustained periods of time, there is a risk of disease outbreaks and the spread of resistant infections. Such events may strain existing sanitation systems or health care facilities if people become ill. Crowding and inadequate facilities contribute to the potential for disease outbreaks (Gautret and Steffen 2016). These events draw people from around the globe and thus may result in the international spread of disease (Gautret and Steffen 2016).

At the same time, many of these events are of great cultural importance and suppression of them is neither a realistic nor a desirable option. There have been extensive discussions of how to address the public health needs of the great numbers of people who undertake pilgrimages or who attend other events that draw great numbers of people together. Vaccination may create herd immunities that reduce risks of disease transmission; for example, for this year's Hajj the Saudi Arabian government is requiring proof of a quadrivalent Meningococcal vaccination in order to receive a visa (Ministry of Hajj 2017). Nonetheless, risks may remain significant for conditions that cannot currently be addressed by vaccination or that are difficult to treat, such as Middle East respiratory syndrome coronavirus (MERS-CoV) or resistant infections. Information too is critical: such well-attended events require imaginative and thoughtful surveillance that informs short-term medical care. Because Saudi Arabia has had the largest number of human cases of MERS-CoV—an estimated 80% (WHO 2017b)—travelers for this year's Hajj are being warned to take extra precautions with respect to sanitation and personal hygiene measures such as handwashing or avoiding direct contact with non-human animals (New Zealand Ministry of Foreign Affairs 2017).

Still other social factors may contribute to the development of resistant disease that can be identified through surveillance. Given the difficulties for women in Saudi Arabia to see physicians without being escorted, it is understandable that in

Saudi Arabia many community pharmacies will dispense antibiotics without a prescription. Zowasi (2016) recommends addressing these issues by increased education especially through social media as to the best approach to respond to the risk of anti-microbial resistant organism.

Still other recommendations about information use involve research on the development of new forms of antimicrobials. According to the most recent review article (Butler et al. 2017), antibiotics "are dramatically undervalued by society, receiving a fraction of the yearly revenue per patient generated by next-generation anticancer drugs." They are in the judgment of these authors an "endangered species,"—but there is some faint encouraging news. WHO and a number of national governments have recently begun to direct attention to the potential threat of resistance and lack of new drugs. Since 2000, five new-in-class antibiotics have been marketed, but these unfortunately only target gram-positive organisms not the gram-negative organisms that are likely to be resistant. Other compounds are also in various stages of the process of clinical trials, but these too are more likely to be active against gram-positive bacteria. In the judgment of the authors of this review article, "the acute positive trend of new approvals masks a chronic underlying malaise in antibiotic discovery and development." Interest in antibiotic development is more likely to be present in smaller biotech companies and in biotech companies located in Europe. The authors conclude: "The only light on the horizon is the continued increase in public and political awareness of the issue." They also observe that with the retrenchment in investment, "we potentially face a generational knowledge gap" and drug development "is now more important than ever."

To address this perilous juncture in antimicrobial research, the Pew Charitable Trust convened a scientific expert group in 2016. The premise of the group was that regulatory challenges, scientific barriers, and diminishing economic returns have led drug companies largely to abandon antibiotic research—yet antimicrobial resistance is accelerating. No entirely new classes of antibiotics useful against resistant organisms have been brought to market that are not derivatives of classes developed before 1984—over 30 years ago. The Pew report advances many explanations for this dismal situation, including importantly the lack of coordinated investment in the relevant basic and translational research. One aspect of the report detailed the major role played by information gaps. Published research is out of date and out of print. Moreover, in today's world of investment in drug discovery, "creating an environment in which data exchange and knowledge sharing are the status quo will be difficult given proprietary concerns and the variety of information types and formats, which may range from historical data to new findings produced as part of this research effort." The Pew consensus is that the following forms of information sharing are needed: a review of what is known about compounds that effectively penetrate gram-negative bacteria, a searchable catalogue of chemical matter including an ongoing list of promising antibacterial compounds, information on screening assays and conditions tested, and an informational database of available biological and physicochemical data. Mechanisms must also be developed for sharing drug discovery knowledge in the area (Pew, pp. 19–20).

In line with Pew, a European antimicrobial resistance project suggests that research is seriously underfunded (Kelly et al. 2015). This group argues that the bulk of the publicly funded research is in therapeutics (63%); among the remainder, 14% of the research was on transmission and only 3% specifically on surveillance. This group also concluded that research is not coordinated and there is little attention to data sharing or sharing of research results. Funding is fragmented, too, with many smaller grants addressing smaller projects independently rather than in a way that builds. This group summarizes: "to conclude, investment at present might not correspond with the burden of antibacterial resistance and the looming health, social, and economic threat it poses on the treatment of infections and on medicine in general. Antibacterial resistance clearly warrants increased and new investment from a range of sources, but improved coordination and collaboration with more informed resource allocation are needed to make a true impact. Hopefully, this analysis will prompt nations to pay due consideration to the existing research landscape when considering future investments."

Additional recommendations from other groups include novel methods for management of resistant disease, such as addressing the intestinal microbiome (e.g. Bassetti et al. 2017); these methods, too, may be furthered by surveillance information as well as information about individual patients.

Analysis of these uses of information from the perspective of vector or victim are, we now argue, incomplete.

The Vector Perspective

When contagious diseases are serious or highly likely to be fatal and treatments for them are limited at best, fear is understandable. Fear may be magnified if the disease is poorly understood, especially until modes of transmission have been identified. Fear may also be magnified if there are no known effective treatments for the disease, as may be the case for extremely drug resistant infections. It is therefore understandable that proposals may come to the fore that emphasize isolation of those who are known to be infected, quarantine of those who have been exposed, or travel bans from areas of known disease outbreaks. Proposals may even include criminalization of those who knowingly or even negligently take risks of infecting others.

All of these possibilities and more were features of the HIV epidemic. Even as understanding of the disease grew and effective treatment became increasingly available, some of these remain. Criminalization of HIV transmission has not waned, despite the many objections raised to it (e.g. Francis and Francis 2013a, b). Although the US ended its immigration ban on HIV+ individuals in 2010, concerns remain about the risks of undiagnosed infections among immigrant populations in the U.S. (Winston and Beckwith 2011) and some countries (for example, Singapore) continue to ban entry for HIV+ travelers planning stays over thirty days (The Global Database 2017).

As epidemic fears have waxed and waned over recent decades, so have imperatives for identifying vectors and constraining their activities. These patterns have been apparent for avian influenza, SARS, Ebola, and Zika, among others. The US still bars entry by non-citizens with a list of conditions including active TB, infectious syphilis, gonorrhea, infectious leprosy, and other conditions designated by Presidential Executive order such as plague or hemorrhagic fevers (CDC 2017).

Indeed, resistant TB has been a frequent illustration of the vector perspective in operation. Multi-drug resistant tuberculosis is transmissible, difficult to treat, and poses a significant public health problem. Its presence can be identified by methods such as testing of sputum samples. When patients are identified with resistant disease, public health authorities may seek to compel treatment or isolation, especially for patients judged unreliable about compliance with treatment. To avoid transmission, public health authorities have proposed isolating patients who have been identified as infected. Because a course of treatment for TB may take many months—and failure to complete the full course may increase the likelihood of resistant disease—isolation may continue for long periods of time. Controversially, during the early 1990s public health officials in New York isolated over 200 patients identified with MDR TB on Roosevelt Island for treatment out of concern that they would be non-compliant with treatment even when they were unlikely to infect others (Coker 2001).

Perhaps one of the most highly publicized events involving a single patient was the odyssey of Andrew Speaker, a lawyer believed to have extremely resistant TB who eluded authorities as he took airplane flights around the globe in the effort to return home. Speaker's journey created an international scare and calls for travel restrictions. Speaker's lawsuit against the Centers for Disease Control and Prevention alleging violations of the federal Privacy Act, he claimed by revealing more information than was necessary for public health purposes, was ultimately resolved on summary judgment for the government, largely because the challenged disclosures had been made by Speaker himself. (*Speaker v. U.S. Department of Health and Human Services Centers for Disease Control and Prevention*, 489 Fed. Appx. 425 (2012); Associated Press 2010) But the saga reveals how individuals perceived as threats may be vilified for what were understandable, if unwise, efforts at self-protection.

WHO travel guidelines provide that individuals known to be infected with resistant TB should not travel until sputum analysis confirms that they are not at risk of disease transmission (WHO 2017). Evidence is limited, however, about the need for this policy. The most recent literature review suggests that risks of transmission during air travel are very low and that there is need for ongoing international collaboration in contact tracing and risk assessment (Kotila et al. 2016). Blanket travel bans encouraging actions that elude detection may reduce, rather than enhance, this needed collaboration. More subtle policies tailored to need would be preferable, but the fears generated by a focus on fear of vectors may make them unlikely to be developed or implemented.

At best, therefore, the vector perspective is incomplete. Focus on it may be counter-productive, if people hide or try to avoid education. It may encourage expenditures on efforts to identify suspected vectors rather than on evidence based efforts to identify risks of transmission and effective modes of prevention. And, of course, it ignores the plight of victims, to which we now turn.

The Victim Perspective

People with resistant infections are not only vectors, they are also victims of disease and have ethical claims to be treated as such (Battin et al. 2007). Indeed, it is likely that vectors will themselves be victims, unless they are carriers of the disease in a manner that does not affect them symptomatically.

Concern for victims may take the form of seeking to ease the burdens of constraints such as isolation. A good illustration of the victim perspective in operation is the WHO publication of a pamphlet on "psychological first aid" to those affected by Ebola. The pamphlet is designed to provide comfort to and meet the basic needs of people infected by Ebola and those who are close to them, while maintained the safety of aids workers (WHO 2014). The recommendations rest on the importance of respect for the dignity of those who are suffering amidst disease outbreaks. It also emphasizes the importance of respect for rights such as confidentiality and non-discrimination. The pamphlet is provisional and designed to be updated as knowledge of safety measures improves; this provisional nature is a recognition of the importance of ongoing development of information about how victims' needs can be safely met.

Despite the concern for victims, foremost in the pamphlet's recommendations is safety, both of aid workers and of disease victims, so that no one is further harmed including victims themselves and others close to them. Overall, the pamphlet attempts to counter impulses to come to the aid of victims that may increase transmission risks, such as unprotected contact with those who are ill. But unexplored tensions remain in the document's recommendations. For example: "Respect privacy and keep personal details of the person's story confidential, if this is appropriate" (p. 22). Nowhere does the document discuss when confidentiality is appropriate or what personal details may be revealed and in what ways. Its manifest and important concern for victims is countered by safety but without discussion of how these goals might be implemented together or reasonably reconciled in practice.

The WHO's most recently-adopted strategy for dealing with health emergencies, the Health Emergencies Programme, provides another illustration of concern for victims that may lie in unexplored tension with other values. The Programme urges cooperative methods to meet the immediate health needs of threatened populations through humanitarian assistance while also addressing causes of vulnerability and recovery (WHO 2016). It is a coordinated strategy for emergency response that will move far beyond merely technical help; WHO describes it as a "profound change for WHO, adding operational capabilities to our traditional technical and normative roles" (WHO 2016). It is aimed to provide crisis help, such as to Hurricane Matthew in Haiti or to areas affected by the Zika virus. It requires a major increase in funding devoted to core emergency efforts. Core funding will come from assessed contributions, flexible contributions that the Director-General has discretion to allocate, and earmarked voluntary contributions. But it is clearly under-funded; WHO reported a 44% funding gap as of October 2016, just to meet the program's core capabilities. Moreover, WHO also reported that it has raised less than a third of the funding needed for the WHO Contingency Fund for Emergencies, a fund deployed for the initial 3 months of an emergency before donor funding becomes available (WHO 2016).

The Health Emergencies Programme reflects reactions to the humanitarian disaster of the Ebola epidemic and criticisms of the WHO level of response. The WHO 2016–2017 budget reflects this response as well (WHO 2015). That budget "demonstrates three strategic shifts" (WHO 2015, p. 2). The first is application of the lessons from Ebola especially the need to strengthen core capacities in preparedness, surveillance and response. The second strategic shift is a focus on universal health coverage, which includes enhancing contributions to maternal and child health, speeding progress towards elimination of malaria, and enhancing work on non-communicable diseases, among other worthy goals. The final strategic shift is towards "emerging threats and priorities"; illustrations of these are "antimicrobial resistance, hepatitis, ageing, and dementia." These are not an obvious group to characterize as "emerging," to the extent that this suggests a developing threat that has not yet become urgent but that may be expected to become so in the near future. Nor are they an obvious group to link together in the same category. This mixture of budgetary priorities suggests is responsiveness to issues raised through consultation with WHO member states, rather than proactive planning.

WHO specific efforts directed to resistance can be characterized as primarily coordination. The WHO website devoted to resistance promotes information sharing and lists research questions and potential funding agencies (WHO 2017a). WHO expresses no judgment about either funding agencies or which of the nearly 100 listed research questions—ranging from research on resistance in day care centers to the biological price that microorganisms pay for resistance—might be fruitfully addressed first or how they might be interconnected.

Concern for victims is surely part of a response to a humanitarian emergency. Responsiveness to urgent health needs is an important goal. Including antimicrobial resistance in a list of "emerging" issues is at least recognition of the problem. But the WHO response to Ebola and the WHO budget overall can be characterized as less than fully set into context in a reasoned way.

Thus, we contend, neither vector nor victim perspectives are adequate. One risks falling prey to fear while the other risks responses that are well-intentioned but that may be difficult to meet or compete with other values in ways that remain underexplored. These perspectives are inevitable and important, but they are each incomplete.

Fairness in Information Use

In our judgment, a primary difficulty with both vector and victim perspectives is that neither are set into context or seen as interconnected. This section suggests how fairness considerations may help in focusing attention to the most pressing questions to ask about antimicrobial resistance and the directions for surveillance and information use to take.

Fairness entered the philosophical lexicon in discussions about justice as procedural, most famously in John Rawls's "Justice as Fairness" (Rawls 1958). As Rawls initially conceptualized his view, it involved a decision procedure for selecting basic principles of justice in which people were unable to gain unfair advantage. As the debates about Rawlsian justice unfolded, a fundamental issue was whether people with radically different capacities and views of the good life could be expected to accept the results of the decision procedure as formulated. Thus critics raised the concern that people with disabilities might be left out of the decision procedure as "non-contributors" to the practice of justice (Nussbaum 2007; Stark 2007). Critics also pressed the argument that people with radically illiberal conceptions of the good would ultimately destabilize the practice of justice in a Rawlsian ideal society (e.g. Williams 2007a, b). Rawls ultimately accepted the point that proceduralism could not yield a universal theory of justice, pulling back his view to the claim that it only represented a vision of justice for a certain kind of liberal society (Rawls 1993).

But fairness also entered the debates about justice in a more substantive way, especially in bioethics. Norman Daniels (1985), for example, expanded a Rawlsian approach to consider justice in health care. The British idea of a "fair innings," in which the opportunities of each to reasonable health over a normal life span are prioritized, was raised particularly with respect to the distribution of health care resources to the elderly (Bognar 2015; Farrant 2009; Harris 1985; Williams 2007b). Like the metaphor of a level playing field, the fair innings argument comes from sports (Francis 2017). It reflects the idea of everyone having a chance to participate in a game that at least gives them a reasonable opportunity for success. There are four aspects of such opportunity: who plays and whether the rules are constructed to give each an opportunity to win that is reasonable are two. Also important is the balance among opportunities to succeed, so that there aren't consistent tilts in one direction or another, as might be characterized by the further metaphor of leveling the playing field. Finally, attention to the interaction between advantages and disadvantages matters, so that participants are encouraged to continue playing the game rather than dropping out.

Our invocation of fairness as a concept is rooted in the judgment that antimicrobial resistance—or other pressing global public health problems, for that matter—exemplify multiple aspects of non-ideal and partial compliance circumstances. Natural circumstances are less than forgiving; new health threats emerge on a regular basis. Antimicrobial resistance is an ongoing natural challenge to effective therapy for deadly diseases. Social circumstances are imperfect, too: overcrowding, poor sanitation, straitened resources for public health and health care, and cultural practices that increase potential for disease transmission all play roles in the development of resistance. Alexander Fleming, the discoverer of penicillin, warned that the development of resistance was likely, but his warning appears not to have been well heard. Finally, efforts to address antimicrobial resistance are riven with noncompliance: over-prescribing by physicians, over-use of antimicrobials in agriculture, individual failures to take medications as prescribed, and concealment of disease out of fear of discovery and persecution. Because the conditions that give rise to these problems of non-compliance may seem urgent—people seeking antimicrobials are in pain or ill, perhaps gravely; people in hiding from health authorities may fear stigmatization or death—they raise in particularly poignant form questions of the extent of obligations under circumstances in which others are not doing what arguably is their fair share (e.g. Stemplowska 2016; Murphy 2000).

Fairness as an ethical concept is especially suited to such imperfect circumstances. It directs attention to how improvements are distributed. Distributions can be more or less fair, if they distribute benefits and burdens in an increasingly inclusive manner (e.g. Francis and Francis 2013a, b). Fairness thus construed is at the heart of perhaps the most influential set of recommendations for ethical pandemic planning, the Canadian *Stand on Guard for Thee* (Toronto Joint Centre 2005). Although much of the discussion of fairness in this document emphasizes inclusive procedures, so that engagement may lead to acceptance of choices as fairly made (e.g., p. 1), the recommendations also contain substantive dimensions. These include fair resource plans for those who fall ill providing necessary services during a pandemic (p. 11) and assurance that people who are affected by choices are reciprocally supported in a way that they do not suffer "unfair economic penalties" (p. 13). Here, the links between fairness and reciprocity are explicit.

These four aspects of fairness—who is included in the play, what opportunities they have, how these opportunities are balanced, and whether there are elements of reciprocity—can be used to set vector and victim perspectives into context in addressing the gathering and use of information about antimicrobial resistance. Over-emphasizing vectors threatens their opportunities and even possible participation. Overemphasizing victims tilts the field unidirectionally, understandably directing resources to immediate need but without consideration of longer-term consequences. Reciprocity may be the most important of all, creating commitment to workable strategies for addressing resistance when there are difficult choices to be made.

Fear, understood as a threat personal health, is often an ally in persuading people to seek preventive care and to change life styles, or to persuade policy makers to create incentives or penalties for decisions that contribute to poor health. But great fear can also lead to immobility. The real threat posed by the rise of antimicrobial resistance does not seem to be easily addressed by a successful alternative in the view of victims or policy makers. Medical personnel are fearful of not responding to the demands of patients for immediate reductions in pain or suffering at relatively low costs. The scale of the threat posed by rapid rise of antimicrobial resistance may be daunting to policy makers especially as funders of research. The cost of developing ever-new generations of antibiotics seems to suggest a great series of short-term solutions especially as pharmaceutical companies respond to incentives to generate near-term profits. In this context, it is worth recalling how the development of the first antimicrobials contributed to more generally shared benefits: when penicillin became known to people as a wonderful drug it actually helped to speed the adoption of the National Health Service in Britain. The popular expectation was health care for all facilitated with the rise of a new generation of low cost wonder drugs and reinforced by low cost vaccinations (Webster 2002). But some of the advantages were short-lived, as the costs of pharmaceuticals grew exponentially and inadequate attention was paid to the risks of overprescribing—once again a cautionary reminder of the importance of emphasizing balance rather than one particular perspective such as victimhood. If a promise of sustaining production at lower costs of ever-new generations of antimicrobials from how information is used can offer benefits more widely, then it becomes easier to impose tougher regulations on antimicrobial use that may to some extent stave off the development of resistance.

This approach in terms of fairness directs attention not only to vectors and to victims seen as separate entities. It also directs attention to how they are often, and unpredictably, twinned—given the epidemiology of resistance spread, it is likely to begin within interlaced communities where vectors are also victims. But it also directs our attention to these issues set in distributive context, raising questions such as these: Who is most likely to be affected by resistance? Who will suffer the most severe consequences from resistance? Who is most likely to be disadvantaged by information gained to counter resistance? Who will suffer the most severe disadvantage? Who will benefit from efforts to counter resistance? How can these benefits be spread more inclusively? And, how are the benefits and burdens of addressing resistance intertwined? Are some primarily beneficiaries, while others are primarily burdened? Are there ways to increase reciprocal linkages in these benefits and burdens, so that efforts to counter resistance are accepted and supported more widely? These are the kinds of questions that need to guide how surveillance is deployed in the effort to counter resistance, not vague generalities about the importance of addressing health infrastructure or bromides about the need to increase resources.

References

Associated Press. 2010. Georgia: Suit against disease centers is revived. *The New York Times* (Oct. 22) [online]. http://www.nytimes.com/2010/10/23/us/23brfs-SUITAGAINSTD_BRF.html.

Bassetti, Matteo, Garyphallia Poulakou, Etienne Ruppe, Emilio Bouza, Sebastian J. Van Hal, and Adrian Brink. 2017. Antimicrobial resistance in the next 30 years, humankind, bugs and drugs: A visionary approach. *Intensive Care Medicine*, epub https://link.springer.com/article/10.1007%2Fs00134-017-4878-x.

Battin, Margaret P., Leslie P. Francis, Jay A. Jacobson, and Charles B. Smith. 2007. *The patient as victim and vector: Ethics and infectious disease*. New York: Oxford University Press.

Bognar, Greg. 2015. Fair innings. *Bioethics* 29 (4): 251–261.

Butler, Mark S., Mark A.T. Blaskovich, and Matthew A. Cooper. 2017. Antibiotics in the clinical pipeline at the end of 2015. *The Journal of Antibiotics* 70: 3024.

Centers for Disease Control and Prevention. 2017. Immigrant and refugee health. https://www.cdc.gov/immigrantrefugeehealth/laws-regs/hiv-ban-removal/final-rule-general-qa.html.

Coker, Richard. 2001. Just coercion? Detention of nonadherent tuberculosis patients. *Annals of the New York Academy of Sciences* 953b: 216–223.

Daniels, Norman. 1985. *Just health care*. 1st ed. New York: Cambridge University Press.

Farrant, Anthony. 2009. The fair innings argument and increasing life spans. *British Medical Journal* 35: 53–56.

Francis, Leslie P. 2017. Promoting equality in and through the paralympics. In *Philosophy: Sport. Macmillan interdisciplinary handbooks*, ed. R. Scott Kretchmar, 245–262. Farmington Hills: Macmillan Reference USA.

Francis, Leslie P., and John G. Francis. 2013a. HIV treatment as prevention: Not an argument for continuing criminalization of HIV transmission. *International Journal of Law in Context* 9 (4): 520–534.

———. 2013b. Informatics and public health surveillance. In *Bioinformatics law: Legal issues for computational biology in the post-genome era*, ed. Jorge Contreras and James Cuticcia. Cleveland: American Bar Association.

Gautret, Philippe, and Robert Steffen. 2016. Communicable diseases as health risks at mass gatherings other than Hajj: What is the evidence? *International Journal of Infectious Diseases* 47: 46–52.

Harris, John. 1985. *The value of life*. London: Routledge & Kegal Paul.

Hoelzer, Karin, Nora Wong, Joe Thomas, Kathy Talkington, Elizabeth Jungman, and Allan Coukell. 2017. Antimicrobial drug use in food-producing animals and associated human health risks: What, and how strong, is the evidence? BMC Veterinary Research 13: 211. https://doi.org/10.1186/s12917-017-1131-3.

Jørgensen, Lars Christian, Sarah Friis Christensen, Gloria Cordoba Currea, Carl Llor, and Lars Bjerrum. 2013. Antibiotic prescribing in patients with acute rhinosinusitis is not in agreement with European recommendations. *Scandinavian Journal of Primary Health Care* 31 (2): 101–105.

Kelly, Ruth, Ghada Zoubiane, Desmond Walsh, Rebecca Ward, and Herman Goossens. 2015. Public funding for research on antibacterial resistance in the JPIAMR countries, the European Commission, and related European Union agencies: A systematic observational analysis. *The Lancet Infectious Diseases* 16 (4): 431–440.

Kotila, S.M., L. Payne Hallström, N. Jansen, P. Helbling, and I. Abubakar. 2016. Review: Systematic review on tuberculosis transmission on aircraft and update of the European Centre for Disease Prevention and Control risk assessment guidelines for tuberculosis transmitted on aircraft (RAGIDA-TB). *Eurosurveillance* 21 (4): 30114. http://www.eurosurveillance.org/ViewArticle.aspx?ArticleId=21357#aff1.

Lam, T.P., and K.F. Lam. 2003. What are the non-biomedical reasons which make family doctors over-prescribe antibiotics for upper respiratory tract infection in a mixed private/public Asian setting? *Journal of Clinical Pharmacy and Therapeutics* 28 (3): 197–201.

Ministry of Hajj, Kingdom of Saudi Arabia. 2017. Saudi Ministry of Health Requirements and Health Matters. http://www.hajinformation.com/main/t20.htm.

Murphy, Liam B. 2000. *Moral demands in nonideal theory*. Oxford: Oxford University Press.

New Zealand Ministry of Foreign Affairs. 2017. Hajj pilgrimage. *Live News* (Aug. 14) [online]. https://livenews.co.nz/2017/08/14/hajj-pilgrimage/.

Nussbaum, Martha C. 2007. *Frontiers of justice: Disability, nationality, species membership*. Cambridge, MA: Harvard University Press.

Rawls, John. 1958. Justice as fairness. *The Philosophical Review* 67 (2): 164–194.

———. 1993. *Political liberalism*. New York: Columbia University Press.

Stark, Cynthia A. 2007. How to include the severely disabled in the contractarian theory of justice. *Journal of Political Philosophy* 15 (2): 127–145.

Stemplowska, Zofia. 2016. Doing more than one's fair share. *Critical Review of International Social and Political Philosophy* 19 (5): 591–608.

The Global Database on HIV-Specific Travel & Residence Restrictions. 2017. Regulations on entry, stay and residence for PLHIV. http://www.hivtravel.org/Default.aspx?PageId=143&Mode=list&StateId=2.

The PEW Charitable Trusts (Pew). 2016. A scientific roadmap for antibiotic discovery. (May 11). http://www.pewtrusts.org/en/research-and-analysis/reports/2016/05/a-scientific-roadmap-for-antibiotic-discovery.

Trap, Birna, and E.H. Hansen. 2002. Treatment of upper respiratory tract infections—A comparative study of dispensing and non-dispensing doctors. *Journal of Clinical Pharmacy and Therapeutics* 27 (4): 289–298.

Unemo, Magnus, Catriona S. Bradshaw, Jane S. Hocking, Henry J. C. de Vries, Suzanna C. Francis, David Mabey, Jeanne M. Marrazzo, Gerard J.B. Sonder, Jane R. Schwebke, Elske Hoornenborg, Rosanna W. Peeling, Susan S. Philip, Nicola Low, & Christopher K. Fairley. 2017. Sexually transmitted infections: challenges ahead. *Lancet Infectious Diseases.* 17(8):e235-e279. 10.1016/S1473-3099(17)30310-9. Epub 9 July 2017.

University of Toronto Joint Centre for Bioethics Pandemic Influenza Working Group (Toronto Joint Centre). 2005. Stand on Guard for Thee: Ethical considerations in preparedness planning for pandemic influenza. http://www.jcb.utoronto.ca/people/documents/upshur_stand_guard.pdf.

Webster, Charles. 2002. *The National Health Service: A political history.* Oxford: Oxford University Press.

WHO. 2005. International Health Regulations, 3rd ed. http://apps.who.int/iris/bitstream/10665/246107/1/9789241580496-eng.pdf?ua=1.

———. 2014. Psychological first aid during Ebola virus disease outbreaks: Provisional version. http://apps.who.int/iris/bitstream/10665/131682/1/9789241548847_eng.pdf?ua=1.

———. 2015. Programme Budget 2016–2017. http://who.int/about/finances-accountability/budget/PB201617_en.pdf.

———. 2016. WHO's new Health Emergencies Programme. http://www.who.int/features/qa/health-emergencies-programme/en/.

———. 2017a. Drug resistance. http://www.who.int/drugresistance/infosharing/en/.

———. 2017b. Middle East respiratory syndrome coronavirus (MERS-CoV) (May). http://www.who.int/mediacentre/factsheets/mers-cov/en/.

Wigton, Robert S., Carol A. Darr, Kitty K. Corbett, Devin R. Nickol, and Ralph Gonzales. 2008. How do community practitioners decide whether to prescribe antibiotics for acute respiratory infections? *Journal of General Internal Medicine* 23: 1615–1620.

Williams, Alan. 2007a. Intergenerational equity: An exploration of the 'fair innings' argument. *Health Economics* 6 (2): 117–132.

Williams, Bernard. 2007b. In *In the beginning was the deed: Realism and moralism in political argument,* ed. Geoffrey Hawthorn. Princeton: Princeton University Press.

Winston, Susanna E., and Curt G. Beckwith. 2011. The impact of removing the immigration ban on HIV-infected persons. *AIDS Patient Care and STDs* 25 (12): 709–711.

World Health Organization (WHO). 2017. International travel and health: Tuberculosis (TB). http://www.who.int/ith/diseases/tb/en/.

Zorgani, Abdulaziz, and Hisham Ziglam. 2013. Letter: Injured Libyan combatant patients: Both vectors and victims of multiresistance bacteria? *Libyan Journal of Medicine* 58: 20325. https://doi.org/10.3402/ljm.v8i0.20325.

Zowasi, Hosam M. 2016. Antimicrobial resistance in Saudi Arabia: An urgent call for an immediate action. *Saudi Medical Journal* 37 (9): 935–940.

9

Solidarity and Antimicrobial Resistance

Søren Holm and Thomas Ploug

Abstract The concept of solidarity has received increasing attention in discussions about public health interventions, both as a possible justification for such interventions and as a possible motivating factors for individual action. This chapter provides an analysis of whether thinking through a lens of solidarity is likely to be helpful in devising strategies and policies to combat antimicrobial resistance. It first provides a critical overview of recent accounts of solidarity and argues that solidarity must be understood as a group based concept. It then applies this conception of solidarity to individual use of antibiotics through a case study of the antibiotic treatment of moderate and severe acne where it is argued that solidarity based thinking is valuable within a context of shared decision-making. Issues of policy making are then discussed and it is argued that basing a policy on solidarity on the one hand constrains the methods chosen to pursue public health goals, but that on the other hand solidarity may provide a strong and durable motivation to comply with such a policy. The limits of solidarity are explored in the final section and it is concluded that 1) the concept of solidarity does have an important role to play in thinking about public health, 2) considerations of solidarity can help us shape the goals and methods of public health policies in the area of antibiotics, and 3) that it is likely that solidarity may also be helpful in thinking through other contentious issues in public health.

Keywords Antibiotic resistance · Bioethics · Collective action · Solidarity

---

S. Holm (✉)
Centre for Social Ethics and Policy, School of Law, University of Manchester, Manchester, UK

Center for Medical Ethics, Faculty of Medicine, University of Oslo, Oslo, Norway
e-mail: soren.holm@manchester.ac.uk

T. Ploug
Centre for Applied Ethics and Philosophy of Science, Department of Communication, Aalborg University, Copenhagen, Denmark
e-mail: ploug@hum.aau.dk

Introduction

Antibiotic resistance in bacteria, viruses and other pathogenic microorganisms is an increasing public health problem. The treatment of infectious diseases depends on the availability of effective antibiotics and modern surgery is only possible because post-operative infections can be effectively treated. It is therefore of the utmost importance to devise policies that can minimise and delay the emergence of resistance, as well as policies that promote the development of new classes of antibiotics.

But developing such policies and ensuring compliance with them is a complicated problem. It is complicated by (1) the fact that the development of resistance is not only caused by misuse or overuse of antibiotics, (2) the possibility of resistant strains and resistance genes to spread rapidly in our globalised and interconnected world, and (3) the close connection between health system deficiencies in resource poor environments and the development of resistance (Daulaire et al. 2015).

Any use of antibiotics can lead to the selection of genetic variants that confer resistance to that antibiotic or class of antibiotics in microorganisms. Although proper use of antibiotics can minimise the emergence of such genetic variants it cannot completely prevent it, and there is some evidence that genes conferring resistance can be present even before the antibiotic is developed and used (Rolo et al. 2017a, b). Patients shed microorganisms during their treatment (e.g. approximately 1×10^{11} bacteria per gram of faeces), and the antibiotics themselves are also excreted in urine and faeces leading to selection for antibiotic resistance in bacteria in the sewer systems of health care institutions (Hansen et al. 2016).

This means that antibiotic resistance cannot be prevented merely by preventing misuse and overuse of antibiotics. In some circumstances we will also need to restrict proper use. We may, for instance have to restrict the use of an effective antibiotic against a known microorganism which is sensitive to that antibiotic in contexts where most of the cases of the illness in question are self-limiting. The cost of this will be that many patients will experience illness for longer than if they had been treated, and that some whose illness turn out not to be self-limiting may suffer more significant effects.

In this paper we will analyse to what extent the concept of 'solidarity' can help in (1) guiding personal and professional decision-making about the use of antibiotics, (2) designing and deciding on proper policies for minimising and delaying the emergence of resistance, and (3) maintaining support for and promoting compliance with anti-resistance policies. Solidarity is an old concept, but has recently experienced a resurgence in public health ethics.

The focus of the paper is on the use of antibiotics in human health care, and primarily on policies that aim to control the use of antibiotics in health care. There are significant issues concerning how to properly incentivise the development of new antibiotics and how to control the marketing of antibiotics, but these issues of 'industrial policy' are better analysed through the concepts of justice and injustice. Antibiotic use in veterinary medicine and in agriculture more generally, e.g. as growth promoters in animal husbandry is also outside the scope of this paper. These practices contribute very significantly to the development and maintenance of antibiotic resistance, but we simply do not have space to analyse them in depth within the solidarity framework.[1]

Solidarity and Public Health

Solidarity is an old concept with roots in both moral theology and socialist/social democratic political philosophy. Both the authors of this paper are from Denmark and up until the mid-1990s 'solidarity talk' was common in Danish political discourse and it is still common within the organised labour movement.

The concept of solidarity has recently been revived in public health ethics by Prainsack & Buyx and by Jennings & Dawson (Dawson and Jennings 2012, Jennings 2015, Jennings and Dawson 2015, Prainsack and Buyx 2011, 2016; see also Baylis et al. 2008).

Prainsack & Buyx develop their conception of solidarity from the bottom up in their important book-length exploration of the concept, building on the concept of the solidaristic act defined in the following way:

> Solidarity is an enacted commitment to carry 'costs' (financial, social, emotional or otherwise) to assist others with whom a person or persons recognise similarity in a relevant aspect. (Prainsack and Buyx 2016, p. 52)

Based on this definition they then distinguish three 'tiers' of solidarity:

1. Interpersonal solidarity
2. Group solidarity
3. Contractual, Legal or Administrative Norms (or perhaps better 'institutionalised solidarity')

And they define group solidarity as:

> … solidarity comprises manifestations of a *shared* commitment to carry costs to assist others with whom people consider themselves bound together through at least one similarity in a relevant respect (e.g. a shared situation, characteristic, or cause). (Prainsack and Buyx 2016, p. 55, emphasis in original)

Other important features of their account are that they see solidarity as an inherently symmetrical relation, and thus distinct from asymmetrical relations like charity (p. 67); and that they claim that solidarity is a hybrid descriptive-normative concepts and that it is therefore "… suited neither to be framed nor applied in the way clearly deontic concepts such as human rights, or justice, can be." (p. 93)

We agree with their analysis in many respects. It is very useful because it shows that although the concept of solidarity has a history which links it historically to socialist and social democratic political philosophy, it can be developed and used

[1] We do not even have space to consider whether or not human networks of solidarity can and should be extended to also encompass some or all animals.

for bioethical purposes without relying on any explicit or implicit socialist premises.[2] However, the commitment to develop the conception from the bottom up, from the individual, isolated solidaristic act leads to some problematic conclusions.

The first problem is that it may not make sense to define a specific class of solidaristic acts without reference to a motive grounded in group solidarity. Acts of beneficence or charity are often based on a recognition of 'similarity in a relevant aspect' between the agent and the beneficiary of the act, e.g. the ability to suffer or the ability to experience a certain kind of welfare benefit or the simple fact that the beneficiary is recognised as being a fellow human being; and beneficial acts based in justice are often built on the recognition that the agent and the recipient are similar in the relevant sense of being moral agents subject to obligations of justice.

The second problem is that it is far from obvious that relations of solidarity are, or have to be inherently symmetrical. Agents may perform solidaristic acts for other persons in the full knowledge that they can perform these acts because they have more power or more resources than those they assist, and that it is unlikely that they will need reciprocation. But, if the acts are motivated by solidarity and not by, for instance pity or a desire to do good works, then they should count as within the scope of solidarity. And even if the acts are performed with the expectation that they will be reciprocated if and when needed, that does not entail that the acts or the relationship is symmetrical at the time when the act is performed. If I, based on a motive of solidarity donate money to the striking workers during a long term strike, I may have an expectation that if ever I was participating in a long term strike someone would, based on solidarity donate money to me and my fellow strikers, but that would not necessarily be an expectation that the money would come from the very same workers who are now on strike, and it could still involve the realisation that I am currently much better off than they are. A strict symmetry requirement would also entail that solidarity with future generations beyond the lifetime of the moral agent would be ruled out, simply because whereas I can do something for future generations, they cannot do anything for me.[3]

It also cannot be definitional for acts of solidarity that they must involve net costs. Walking in the 1st of May parade with the other members of the blacksmiths' labour union was, at least in years when the weather was good, a great source of joy for one of our grandfathers, but it was also an act of solidarity and identification with the union, its members and its causes, as well as with the larger network of labour unions.

Jennings & Dawson has a more traditional understanding of solidarity as a group concept and identify three relational dimensions of solidarity:

> The fundamental gesture or posture of solidarity is *standing up beside*. This posture has three relational dimensions: standing up *for*, standing up *with*, and standing up *as*. (p.32, emphasis in original)

---

[2] Whether that is sufficient to ensure that those socialist historical connotations will not be activated in the minds of readers or listeners when the term 'solidarity' is used is a different question.

[3] Except, perhaps keeping my good reputation alive.

We stand up for when we "assist or advocate for the other" (p 36). We stand up with when our solidarity requires us to enter "into the lifeworld of the other"; and we stand up as when there is "a yet stronger degree of identification between the agents of solidaristic support and the recipients of such support." (p. 37). These three dimensions are not fundamentally different types of solidarity and they all draw their justification from the same conception of solidarity, but they point to different levels of engagement and action. It is, for instance uncontroversial that health care professionals should in many circumstances stand up for the patient groups they serve, but their obligation to stand up with these patient groups only get activated in certain contexts, and it is perhaps even rarer that they are required to stand up as with a patient group. But, the obligation to stand up as may be activated in more circumstances for health care professionals if the issue that requires solidaristic action is an issue affecting other health care professionals. In our analyses below of the implications of solidarity for individual and group actions and societal policies in relation to antimicrobial resistance we use Jennings & Dawson's three dimensions to indicate the level of engagement and commitment necessary for a particular kind of solidarity based action or policy to be likely to be effective.

Solidarity and Antimicrobial Resistance

Antimicrobial resistance is a problem that may potentially affect each and every one of us. It may currently be a more significant problem in some areas of the world, but it is not geographically containable. In order to reduce the rate at which antimicrobial resistance develops and spreads we also all have to be involved, since there is no use of antibiotics which does not promote resistance to some small degree.

We thus have a coordination problem. Each of us will in each instance where antibiotics can be prescribed personally benefit or potentially benefit by using antibiotics more than is optimal seen from the point of an optimal, overall balance between use and development of resistance. Or to put it the other way around, slowing down the development of resistance will require each of us sometimes to suffer when that suffering could have been potentially reduced by the prescription of antibiotics.

Coordination problems can, as discussed in other chapters of this book be solved in a variety of different ways, e.g. by changing the choice architecture and/or incentive structure. But some of these more structural solutions may either be illiberal in the sense that they reduce the option space available to individuals, even if none of the individual choices have any harmful consequences as individual choices, or they may create perverse incentives to try to circumvent restrictions in the choice architecture. It is therefore worth considering whether there are alternative options.

Can considerations of solidarity help to solve these coordination problems in a more constructive way, and what is required for solidarity to be activated?

If we look at Jennings & Dawson's three relational dimensions of solidarity it seems to be the case that even persons who have not realised that antimicrobial resistance is a problem for themselves can come to see that they ought to stand up for others in relation to antimicrobial resistance. They might, for instance decide to stand up for victims of extensively drug-resistant tuberculosis (XDR-TB) in sub-Saharan Africa, because they recognise some connection between themselves and the victims, even though they do not see themselves in any way threatened by XDR-TB.

However, once persons have realised that they share in the problem of antimicrobial resistance the two more intensely relational dimensions of solidarity can be activated, i.e. they can come to the realisation that they have to stand up with or as those who are threatened by antimicrobial resistance.

This does, potentially have different implications for ordinary persons /patients and for health care professionals. Ordinary persons can stand up with others in a number of ways in this context, they can advocate for policy changes, for research investment and for increased health care; and they can stand up as and take responsibility for their own use of antibiotics and encouraging others to do the same.

Health care professionals have a wider range of actions available to them because of their roles as gatekeepers to antibiotics, experts in public debates, and trusted advisors to individual patients. But this also means that they have to bring two different perspectives to bear, their personal perspective and their professional perspective; and that they can be part of potentially different networks of solidarity (e.g. solidarity with other health care professionals in areas of the world where resistance is very prevalent).

It is important to note that activating solidarity in the context of antimicrobial resistance does not necessarily have to be based solely on the realisation that I and others share this particular similarity or vulnerability. Groups within which we feel and enact solidarity are often sustained by multiple, complexly intertwined perceived similarities (e.g. a national, regional or professional identity that engenders group solidarity is not just about one shared feature), and it may well be that the chance of successfully engendering 'antimicrobial solidarity' is much larger if it takes place within already existing networks of solidarity. Single similarity solidarity may in some instances be strong, but multi-similarity solidarity is often stronger, partly because it receives support from a multiplicity of motivating factors.

It is likely that the most important and effective kind of solidaristic identification and action in relation to antimicrobial resistance is if enough people stand up as and take responsibility for their own use of antibiotics. What are the necessary conditions for this kind of solidarity to be engendered and for it to spread within already existing networks of solidarity? The first necessary precondition is, as mentioned above the realisation that antimicrobial resistance is not only a problem for others, it is also a problem for me and for others like me. However, for this to result in more than a sentiment of solidarity or a solidarity based call or activism for others to do something, I also need to know that there is something I can do personally in relation to the use of antibiotics. Many people in the industrialised world have probably internalised three key messages about antibiotics during their own upbringing, and later as parents:

1. Don't ask for antibiotics unnecessarily, e.g. when there is no bacterial infection
2. Take the antibiotics if they are offered by the doctor
3. Take the full course of antibiotics that is prescribed

1. and 3. were traditionally backed up by the claim that this will help prevent the development of resistance, and 2. by the general idea that if a doctor offers a treatment option it must be good for you. However, 3. which has been a mainstay of antibiotic folk-knowledge for generations has now been repudiated by a group of scientist in a recent high profile paper where they claim that taking the full course actually promotes the development of resistance (Llewelyn et al. 2017).

So, what knowledge do people now need to have in order to be able to act effectively in this context? They should still not ask for antibiotics when they are not necessary, but the concept of 'not necessary' may have to be further explicated so that we all understand that many bacterial infections are self-limiting and therefore not in need of antibiotic treatment, and also that pursuing treatment even when it is technically effective may bring about bad consequences for others to which we stand in a relation of solidarity.

Let us briefly analyse a specific case study of antibiotic use through the lens of solidarity, i.e. the use of antibiotics in the treatment of acne (Acne vulgaris) in teenagers and adolescents. Acne is a common disease and moderate and severe acne can lead to permanent scarring of the skin, as well as social and psychological problems in those affected by the condition (Hassan et al. 2009; Kellett and Gawkrodger 1999; Murray and Rhodes 2005). Oral antibiotics have for decades been used when topical treatments have been tried but turn out not to be effective and before the prescription of systemic isotretinoin or other retinoic acid analogues, since the retinoic acid analogues have many and potentially severe side-effects (Nagler et al. 2016). There has, however been an increasing realisation that whilst this use of oral antibiotics is effective in many cases, it also leads to increasing antimicrobial resistance (Dreno et al. 2014; Sinnott et al. 2016). What implications do solidarity in terms of standing up with and as have for patients and doctors in this scenario? We will first focus on the patient-doctor encounter and then move on to the question of policy.

In the patient-doctor encounter the enactment of solidarity is a matter for personal and potentially shared decision-making. The doctor can and should advise the patient on the benefits and drawbacks of antibiotics and of other available treatments and the patient should make a decision based on an evaluation of how the different treatment options will affect his or her life and life plans. What solidarity brings to the table are two things, it provides the doctor with a license (and potential obligation) to appeal to the patients solidaristic motivations and it creates an obligation for the patient to consider the choice through the lens of solidarity and not merely as an individual decision. This does not mean that the patient has to refuse antibiotics, or that the doctor has not to mention them as one of the treatment options. Acne is not a trivial disease, the side-effects of other available treatments are significant, and it is only the patient who can judge whether the sacrifice of forgoing antibiotics is outweighed by the solidaristic public health benefits in terms of reducing the development of antibiotic resistance. It is also important to note that the doctor's license to appeal to solidaristic motivations is not generated by the doctor's professional role but by the fact that he or she stands with the patient in a mutual relation of solidarity and that they both recognise this.

Things are more complicated at the policy level. The 'spontaneous' enactment of solidarity that we would wish to crystallise in policy arise in a situation where the doctor interpellates the patient as a person within a network of solidarity and encourages the patient to consider and enact solidarity in his or her decision-making, and where the patient enacts solidarity in a nuanced way by giving proper weight to the public health consequences of using antibiotics in his or her specific circumstances. This is tricky to implement as a policy and the main risks are that the doctor will be seen not as someone who stands with the patient and interpellates him or her in a network of solidarity, but as an agent of the state or the public health system, and that the patient will therefore not engage in solidaristic decision-making but perceive the situation as one where he or she is simply being asked or forced to sacrifice personal interests for some abstract conception of the public good. To avoid this problem the justification given for a policy, the way it is communicated to doctors and patients, and the way in which it is being implemented in health care will have to foreground solidarity considerations as the driving force behind the policy. A policy of simply banning the use of oral antibiotics for the treatment of acne is, for instance unlikely to sustain a solidarity based motivation for compliance.

Consideration of the implications of solidarity can also guide the choice of methods used to pursue public health goals in other areas. It has for instance been suggested in the literature that the active stigmatisation of the overweight and obese is an acceptable public health intervention, if there is evidence that it is effective (Callahan 2013); and there have been suggestions that targeted stigmatisation of farmers whose pigs carry multi-resistant bacteria is acceptable or perhaps even appropriate.[4] But, if there are some obese people or some pig farmers within my circles of solidarity a choice of pursuing active stigmatisation to further public health goals becomes potentially problematic seen from the perspective of solidarity. These are people with whom I share important things and with whom I work on common projects and not people who should be harmed or ridiculed. And, given that standing up with or as them requires me to understand their lifeworld I may well come to understand why they act as they do. More generally considerations of solidarity enjoin us to choose supportive methods in our public health policies, and only resort to proscription when absolutely necessary.

[4] For a rejection of this view on other grounds than solidarity see Ploug et al. 2015.

Solidarity as a Motivational Factor

We have argued above that considerations of solidarity can be useful in the design of policies to minimise and delay antibiotic resistance. But, building on the case study we need to consider solidarity as a motivating factor for action in more detail. We do not want to become embroiled in the interminable discussion about whether moral considerations necessarily motivate, or whether they only motivate when combined with a suitable desire. And, working with a concept like solidarity we do not need to become embroiled in that debate because realising that one has an obligation derived from or in solidarity straddles the cognitive/affective divide. Being in a relation of solidarity with a group is not a purely cognitive matter, but also a matter of felt identification. You don't walk in the parade on the eighth of March, or participate in a 'Reclaim the Streets' action purely on the basis of a dispassionate, rational assessment of your ethical obligations. You do it because you identify with the cause and with the group pursuing the cause.

This motivating force of solidarity lead to and support individual solidaristic action, but it can also be an important factor in engendering support for policy change and maintaining support for policies once they are implemented. However, the mere fact that a policy builds on or crystallises an already existing, or a developing solidarity based practice does not automatically mean that the support will transfer from the practice to the new context where what was previously a freely chosen action is now prescribed and must be performed (or proscribed and no longer available).

In the design of policies we therefore need to be careful not to lose the connection to solidarity as a motivating factor. The policy in a sense has to continue to speak to people and call them out in the language of solidarity and interpellate them as active participants in networks of solidarity.

This has implication both for how policies should be designed and how they should be communicated. We need to understand which networks of solidarity the relevant groups of citizens are embedded within, and design policies that appeal to those already existing networks.

The Extent and Limitations of Solidarity

There are a number of possible criticisms of the line of argument which has been pursued above. Here we want to look at two of them which are especially relevant in the context of antibiotic resistance since it is a global problem that needs global solutions.

The first possible criticism is that because we develop solidarity as a group concept, there will be some individuals and groups that are outside the solidarity group, that are Other than the ones included in our solidarity and who will be disadvantaged by solidarity in the in-group. The second criticism is that it is implausible to think that the solidarity of ordinary people could ever have a global scope (Holm 1993). Saints may aspire to global solidarity, but most of us restrict our solidarity to smaller and more local groups. Taken together these two criticisms imply that solidarity is an unsuitable, and perhaps even pernicious concept on which to base a solution to a global public health problem.

We take the second criticism to be empirically true. Few people manage to engender a state of 'solidarity with the people of the world'[5] in themselves (*pace* West-Oram and Buyx 2017). But perhaps that is not what is needed for solidarity to have global reach and be useful in supporting public health policies and initiatives. A global reach of local solidarity can come about in two ways. The simplest way is if local networks of solidarity are exhaustive in the sense that everyone is a member of at least one local network of solidarity, and if the results of solidarity in all, or perhaps just most of these networks contribute to a similar aim, i.e. in the present context the conservation of effective antibiotics through a reduction in the development of resistance. In this scenario a positive global outcome can be achieved by purely local action. Each local network of solidarity does not have to pursue an aim which is precisely identical to that of other networks. The second way in which local solidarity can have global reach is when we have local, but overlapping circles of solidarity that reach in an unbroken chain from people in the affluent north to people in the impoverished south. This may be sufficient to sustain the public health policies globally. In such a situation, persons may for instance accept policies restricting the use of antibiotics based on their solidarity with their fellow citizens in a particular country or region, but most of the people in that circle of solidarity which is defined by local citizenship will also be in other overlapping circles of solidarity based on other identifications like language, gender, profession etc. etc. Some of these overlapping circles may reach directly from the north to the south, there may for instance be solidarity among nurses or teachers or solidarity based on shared history. Others may be longer and involve more linking circles of solidarity but may never the less still be effective.

The first criticism also contains an element of truth, but it is perhaps not as damaging to the use of solidarity as it initially seems. It is undoubtedly true that there are some circles of solidarity that are partly constituted by identifying a particular group of others as 'the enemy', or as the radical Other. Communist solidarity among workers for instance posits the violent struggle between the working class and the capitalist class as an inevitable historical fact. However, not all forms of solidarity have to work in that way, and most do not. Danish identity and solidarity among Danes, for instance originally relied on distinguishing Danes from Swedes and Germans and seeing those two groups as enemies. But, although Swedes and Germans are still the Other and instantiate all of the traits that are non-Danish and therefore not-ours, they are no longer the enemy. So whereas solidarity almost inevitably expresses a form of partiality, which is partly what distinguishes it from thin

[5] 'Solidaritet med verdens folk' is a common slogan in left wing politics in the Nordic countries

conceptualisations of justice or utility maximisation, it may be a perfectly benign type of partiality.[6]

Conclusion

In this paper we have argued for three main conclusions. First, that the concept of solidarity has an important role to play in analysing how individuals and groups can and should act in relation to the threat of antimicrobial resistances and that it is an important counterweight to pure self-interest. Second, that considerations of solidarity can help us to shape both the goals and the methods of public health policies in order to make them long-term socially sustainable. And, third by implication that given that solidarity is helpful when thinking through one thorny issue in public health ethics and policy, it is likely to be helpful in other areas of public health ethics as well and that it therefore warrants continued attention from the public health (ethics) community.

We have also analysed the problems in moving from a voluntary practice sustained by solidarity to an official policy crystallising that practice as prescriptions and proscriptions and shown that careful design and communication is necessary not to lose the motivating force of solidarity when formulating policy.

References

Baylis, F., N.P. Kenny, and S. Sherwin. 2008. A relational account of public health ethics. *Public Health Ethics* 1 (3): 196–209.

Callahan, D. 2013. Obesity: Chasing an elusive epidemic. *Hastings Center Report* 43 (1): 34–40.

Daulaire, N., A. Bang, G. Tomson, J.N. Kalyango, and O. Cars. 2015. Universal access to effective antibiotics is essential for tackling antibiotic resistance. *The Journal of Law, Medicine & Ethics* 43 (S3): 17–21.

Dawson, A., and B. Jennings. 2012. The place of solidarity in public health ethics. *Public Health Reviews* 34 (1): 65–79.

Dreno, B., D. Thiboutot, H. Gollnick, V. Bettoli, S. Kang, J.J. Leyden, A. Shalita, and V. Torres. 2014. Antibiotic stewardship in dermatology: Limiting antibiotic use in acne. *European Journal of Dermatology* 24 (3): 330–334.

Hansen, T.A., T. Joshi, A.R. Larsen, P.S. Andersen, K. Harms, S. Mollerup, E. Willerslev, K. Fuursted, L.P. Nielsen, and A.J. Hansen. 2016. Vancomycin gene selection in the microbiome of urban Rattus norvegicus from hospital environment. *Evolution, Medicine, and Public Health* 2016 (1): 219–226.

Hassan, J., S. Grogan, D. Clark-Carter, H. Richards, and V.M. Yates. 2009. The individual health burden of acne: Appearance-related distress in male and female adolescents and adults with back, chest and facial acne. *Journal of Health Psychology* 14 (8): 1105–1118.

[6] We will here assume without argument that any complete system of ethics for human agents must incorporate various types of partiality.

Holm, S. 1993. Solidarity, justice and health care priorities. In *Solidarity, justice and health care priorities*, Health service studies, ed. Z. Szawarski and D. Evans, vol. 8, 53–64. Linköping: Linköping University Press.

Jennings, B. 2015. Relational liberty revisited: Membership, solidarity and a public health ethics of place. *Public Health Ethics* 8 (1): 7–17.

Jennings, B., and A. Dawson. 2015. Solidarity in the moral imagination of bioethics. *Hastings Center Report* 45 (5): 31–38.

Kellett, S.C., and D.J. Gawkrodger. 1999. The psychological and emotional impact of acne and the effect of treatment with isotretinoin. *British Journal of Dermatology* 140 (2): 273–282.

Llewelyn, M.J., J.M. Fitzpatrick, E. Darwin, C. Gorton, J. Paul, T.E.A. Peto, L. Yardley, S. Hopkins, and A.S. Walker. 2017. The antibiotic course has had its day. *BMJ* 358: j3418.

Murray, C.D., and K. Rhodes. 2005. Nobody likes damaged goods: The experience of adult visible acne. *British Journal of Health Psychology* 10 (2): 183–202.

Nagler, A.R., E.C. Milam, and S.J. Orlow. 2016. The use of oral antibiotics before isotretinoin therapy in patients with acne. *Journal of the American Academy of Dermatology* 74 (2): 273–279.

Ploug, T., S. Holm, and M. Gjerris. 2015. The stigmatization dilemma in public health policy-the case of MRSA in Denmark. *BMC Public Health* 15 (1): 640.

Prainsack, B., and A. Buyx. 2011. *Solidarity: Reflections on an emerging concept in bioethics*. London: Nuffield Council on Bioethics.

———. 2016. *Solidarity in biomedicine and beyond*. Cambridge: Cambridge University Press.

Rolo, J., P. Worning, J.B. Nielsen, R. Bowden, O. Bouchami, P. Damborg, L. Guardabassi, et al. 2017a. Evolutionary origin of the staphylococcal cassette chromosome mec (SCCmec). *Antimicrobial Agents and Chemotherapy* 61 (6): e02302–e02316.

Rolo, J., P. Worning, J.B. Nielsen, R. Sobral, R. Bowden, O. Bouchami, P. Damborg, et al. 2017b. Evidence for the evolutionary steps leading to mecA-mediated β-lactam resistance in staphylococci. *PLoS Genetics* 13 (4): e1006674.

Sinnott, S.-J., K. Bhate, D.J. Margolis, and S.M. Langan. 2016. Antibiotics and acne: An emerging iceberg of antibiotic resistance? *British Journal of Dermatology* 175 (6): 1127–1128.

West-Oram, P.G., and A. Buyx. 2017. Global health solidarity. *Public Health Ethics* 10 (2): 212–224.

10

Justifying Antibiotic Resistance Interventions: Uncertainty, Precaution and Ethics

Niels Nijsingh, D. G. Joakim Larsson, Karl de Fine Licht, and Christian Munthe

Abstract This chapter charts and critically analyses the ethical challenge of assessing how much (and what kind of) evidence is required for the justification of interventions in response antibiotic resistance (ABR), as well as other major public health threats. Our ambition here is to identify and briefly discuss main issues, and

N. Nijsingh (✉)
Centre for Antibiotic Resistance Research (CARe), University of Gothenburg, Gothenburg, Sweden

Department of Philosophy, Linguistics and Theory of Science (FLoV), University of Gothenburg, Gothenburg, Sweden

Institute of Ethics, History and Theory of Medicine, Ludwig Maximilians Universität, Munich, Germany
e-mail: niels.nijsingh@med.uni-muenchen.de

D. G. J. Larsson
Centre for Antibiotic Resistance Research (CARe), University of Gothenburg, Gothenburg, Sweden

Department of Infectious Diseases, Institute of Biomedicine, The Sahlgrenska Academy, University of Gothenburg, Gothenburg, Sweden
e-mail: joakim.larsson@fysiologi.gu.se

K. de Fine Licht
Centre for Antibiotic Resistance Research (CARe), University of Gothenburg, Gothenburg, Sweden

Department of Technology Management and Economics, Chalmers University of Technology, Gothenburg, Sweden
e-mail: karl.licht@sp.se

C. Munthe
Centre for Antibiotic Resistance Research (CARe), University of Gothenburg, Gothenburg, Sweden

Department of Philosophy, Linguistics and Theory of Science (FLoV), University of Gothenburg, Gothenburg, Sweden
e-mail: christian.munthe@gu.se

point to ways in which these need to be further advanced in future research. This will result in a tentative map of complications, underlying problems and possible challenges. This map illustrates that the ethical challenges in this area are much more complex and profound than is usually acknowledged, leaving no tentatively plausible intervention package free of downsides. This creates potentially overwhelming theoretical conundrums when trying to justify what to do. We therefore end by pointing out two general features of the complexity we find to be of particular importance, and a tentative suggestion for how to create a theoretical basis for further analysis.

Keywords Antibiotic resistance · Public health ethics · Precautionary principle · Complexity

Antibiotic Resistance

Antibiotic resistance is emerging as one of our largest global challenges: more and more bacterial infections[1] are becoming increasingly impervious to antibiotics, which increases morbidity, mortality and societal costs around the world.

The evolutionary principle that drives ABR is relatively simple: when populations of bacteria are exposed to an antibiotic, strains that have acquired resistance to the drug (through mutations or through uptake of genetic material) are favoured over the sensitive ones. The emergence of ABR on a macro-scale is, however, notoriously complex.[2] One reason is that ABR is a global phenomenon with a variety of causes on different levels and in different contexts, some of which are poorly understood.

The most obvious cause of ABR is the use of antibiotics in humans, especially when antibiotics are used inappropriately (e.g. when overly broad antibiotics are used, or when a patient has no benefit from antibiotic treatment). The use of antibiotics in animals, both for treatment and prevention of disease and for growth promotion, also contributes to the problem.[3] Some bacteria have the ability to colonize both humans and domestic animals, and mobile genetic elements, such as resistance plasmids, often move across bacterial species. Hence, there are no firm barriers that

---

[1] We will limit ourselves here to antibiotic resistance. Antibiotic resistance is a sub-category of antimicrobial resistance, which also includes drug resistance in viruses, fungi and other microorganisms than bacteria.

[2] World Health Organization (2014). *The evolving threat of antimicrobial resistance: options for action*. Geneva, Switzerland: World Health Organization.

[3] Anomaly, J. (2020). Antibiotics and Animal Agriculture; The Need for Global Collective Action. In Ethics and Drug Resistance: Collective Responsibility for Global Public Health. Springer, Cham.

separate the microflora of animals from that of humans. The external environment is another source of resistance, both as a transmission route for certain pathogens, for example through faecal contamination of water, and as a source for resistance genes that over time are recruited from harmless bacteria into pathogens, assisted by a selection pressure from antibiotics.[4] The need to take into account the interconnection between humans, animals and the external environment is often referred to as a "One Health perspective".[5]

Clearly, there is an urgent need to address all of these causes of ABR and implement interventions at different sites and different levels of organization. However, as we will see, securing the evidence required to establish both the effectiveness and the risks of such interventions, comes at a moral price. This raises in a straightforward manner the question of what the criteria of evidence should be for the various interventions that aim to fight ABR. This question links the ethical justification of ABR interventions to debates around the ethics of risk and precaution. In other words, all ABR interventions pose the challenge of what quality of evidence for what balance of risks and possible benefits is required for such an intervention to be justified.

Precaution

The notion of precaution is central to much public health and environmental thinking. Specifically, when faced with complex and potentially extremely threatening phenomena such as a pandemic, global warming or pollution, it makes sense both to act in response to them even if there is a lack of evidence, but also to proceed with caution when enacting precautionary measures to mitigate or prevent damage.

Scholars of the *Precautionary Principle* (PP) have worked to express this intuition more clearly, resulting in a generic criterion of justified decision-making and policy arrangements that can be expressed in the following way:

> *... in the face of an activity that may produce great harm, we (or society) have reason to ensure that the activity is not undertaken, unless it has been shown not to impose too serious risks.*[6]

This criterion expresses three basic things: First, the idea that uncertain major threats may provide reason for action.[7] Second, the contention that whatever such

---

[4] Bengtsson-Palme, Johan, and DG Joakim Larsson (2015). Antibiotic resistance genes in the environment: prioritizing risks. *Nature Reviews Microbiology* 13.6: 396–396.

[5] Boden, L. & D. Mellor. (2020). Epidemiology and ethics of antimicrobial resistance in animals. In Ethics and Drug Resistance: Collective Responsibility for Global Public Health. Springer, Cham.

[6] Munthe, Christian (2016). Precautionary principle. In: Ten Have (ed.) *Encyclopedia of global bioethics*. Dordrecht: Springer International Publishing.

[7] Compare also: "uncertainty should not be a reason for inaction in the face of serious environmental threats". Daniel Steel calls this idea the ´meta-precautionary principle´. Note that the vagueness of this procedural meta-criterion allows PP to be applied in a large number of different contexts

actions are taken must not themselves impose too serious risks or new uncertain major threats, and, third, that we are required to *demonstrate reasons* both why responses to threats are motivated and why apparent threats may be accepted. The criterion expresses a generic formula, within which more specific PP *versions*, or specific precautionary policy suggestions, must fit in order to be justified. There are thus various ways to flesh out the idea that we have reason to take precautions in the face of major, but uncertain threats. As a version of PP is specified, it further delineates what can properly be considered *responsible* decision-making in such contexts, not least regarding what is required more precisely to satisfy the requirement of demonstrating reasons for whatever precautionary action is suggested.[8]

One basic assumption underlying PP is that there is a moral price to exposing people to risk, as well as to proceed with activities in the face of uncertain risks. However, there is also always a price to any precautionary intervention that aims to clarify uncertainties and to prevent or mitigate risks: these will always claim resources that could have been used for other worthwhile purposes, create risks of their own, and delay or stop possibly valuable activities. For that reason, suggestions for precautionary action need to be subjected to precautionary scrutiny too, and to be justified it needs to be demonstrated that they incur an acceptable price and level of precaution. Particularly in systemically complex situations, the emergence of risks and uncertainties on various levels raises complications concerning how to balance the type and severity of the various harms and uncertainties involved.

A version of PP has to set *standards* concerning when precautionary action is required, and what is required of it in order to be responsible. Daniel Steel has recently explained this in terms of a ‘tripod’, consisting of a knowledge condition, a harm condition, and a suggested precautionary action.[9] Variations of how this tripod is construed will affect the price of precaution, as well as the level of precaution enacted. A PP version thus needs to specify for (1) any suggested precautionary action, (2) what threat is sufficiently serious for such action to be defensible, and (3) what degree of uncertainty is acceptable for it. For example, in order to, say, justify taking expensive precautionary measures to curb ABR (1), there needs to be a scientifically plausible model (3) in which failure to introduce these measures leads to significant economic or health damage (2). Whether or not in a specific case the model leading to harm is ´plausible´ and the damage is ´significant´ of course requires further elaboration. In any justifiable specification of the ‘tripod’, it is necessary to balance in a responsible way the need for precautionary action against the price of precaution.

Although details vary among authors, critical debate on what it takes to justify a PP version has led to a reasonably broad consensus on some minimal desiderata. These regard that a sound PP must not balance its required level and price of

---

and on different levels of organization. See Steel, Daniel (2014). *Philosophy and the precautionary principle*. Cambridge University Press.

[8] Munthe, Christian (2011). *The price of precaution and the ethics of risk*. Dordrecht: Springer.

[9] Steel (2014).

precaution *arbitrarily* (but according to a general principle that applies equally to all cases), that it needs to avoid so-called *precautionary paradox*, and that principle for responsible balancing of precautionary level and price must be *proportional*.[10]

PP is *arbitrary* when it offers no good, generalizable reasons why a specific course of action is acceptable or not. If an appeal to PP is used to recommend intervention 1, but to prohibit intervention 2, it should be able to meaningfully distinguish between the two measures and show how these are relevantly different. Note that the requirement to avoid arbitrariness also excludes treating the *status quo* with special regard: the fact that things are currently done in certain way is not in itself an argument for doing it that way.[11] It also means that whatever requirements are set by the specification of the tripod in a PP, these apply both to uncertain threats in order to justify precautionary action, *and* to the uncertainties of these actions themselves.

This links to the need to avoid 'precautionary paradox'. PP can lead to paradox in two related ways: Either its requirements are so strong that it tends to ban all options in most situations, thereby undermining any capacity to guide decision-making.[12] Or it issues inconsistent prescriptions by requiring and banning one and the same option.[13] It has been a theme among critics to point out how simplistic versions of PP may easily become paradoxical in any or both of these ways.[14]

The desideratum of proportionality follows from both of these requirements. In order to avoid paradox and arbitrariness, a justified version of PP must present a principle of responsible balancing of what level of precaution is required and what price of precaution is acceptable to pay that applies equally to all situations, as well as to all options in such situations. Any plausible version of PP will thus offer principled grounds for comparing suggested precautionary interventions, or the acceptance of an uncertainty or a threat, to alternative options in a unified manner. Such a version will express an allegedly morally responsible way of balancing the required level and price of precaution. To justify a specific precautionary action in a situation, it is therefore necessary to point how such a PP version supports it. As different situations vary with regard to what options are available, what stakes in terms of threats and prospects these actualise, and what knowledge is available with regard to these factors, one and the same precautionary intervention may therefore be

[10] Munthe, 2011, 2016; Munthe, C. (2017). *Precaution and Ethics: Handling risks, uncertainties and knowledge gaps in the regulation of new biotechnologies*. Berne: Swiss Federal Office for Buildings and Publications and Logistics (FOBL); Steel, (2014).

[11] However, there may be good instrumental reasons to be cautious when implementing change in a situation of great uncertainty. We will return to that point later.

[12] What Munthe (2011, ch. 2) has called *decisional paralysis*.

[13] What Steel (2014) terms *inconsistency*.

[14] Holm, Søren, and John Harris (1999). "Precautionary principle stifles discovery." Nature 400.6743: 398–398. Sunstein, Cass R (2005). *Laws of fear: Beyond the precautionary principle*. Cambridge University Press. McKinney, WJ, & Hill, HH (2000). Of sustainability and precaution: The logical, epistemological, and moral problems of the precautionary principle and their implications for sustainable development. *Ethics and the Environment*, 5: 77–87.

justifiable in some situations, but not in others. This regards also what quality and type of information about risks and effectiveness we require, and how much of further investigation to mitigate uncertainties is needed in the light of that. Precautionary requirements will therefore be gradual rather than absolute, and context-dependent rather than rigid. Different situations will justify different levels of precaution, and different prices of precaution to attain such levels.[15]

This regards not least the option of postponing a specific intervention in order to gather more evidence to ensure its effectiveness and responsibility. Possibly, this is the most common type of precautionary measure, familiar from standard regulation of drugs and the introduction of novel biotechnology.[16] It is also easy to see how this type of precautionary action may often be justified on the basis of a defensible version of PP. However, knowledge is never perfect, and the option to further update the basis of information for assessing the effectiveness and riskiness of an intervention is ever present. So, when do we know enough? How much time and resources should we spend on making sure that what we do in order to invoke responsible precautionary response to dangers and uncertainties will not in fact worsen the situation from a precautionary standpoint by invoking an unjustifiable price of precaution? This is a distinct ethical issue that becomes a particular challenge in the face of complex and drastic public health threats, such as ABR, where the price of delaying interventions is obvious, and costs and new risks of conducting research are salient. If we wait, the ABR problem continues to grow and increasingly threatens to overwhelm us, and if we experiment with interventions this will usually create new uncertainties and risks of harm. At the same time, unproven interventions may both escalate the ABR problem, and expand it to include severe policy failures. This takes us to the question of how these stakes, and options of collecting (or not collecting) evidence, should be assessed and evaluated.

Evidence

Traditionally, guidelines for evidence basing and research in the area of medicine confine themselves to clinical trials of biomedical interventions, focusing mostly on the immediate somatic effects on individual patients.[17] At the same time, as mentioned, ABR (and most other public health) interventions greatly surpass that area, and mostly occur outside of immediate therapeutic action (although sometimes intended to affect it, e.g., those interventions that regard antibiotic prescription practices). However, the recently revised guidelines by the Council for International Organizations of Medical Sciences (CIOMS) allow for a broader conception of

[15] Munthe, (2017).

[16] Munthe (2011), p. 97. See also Munthe, (2017).

[17] World Medical Association (2014). "World Medical Association Declaration of Helsinki: ethical principles for medical research involving human subjects." *The Journal of the American College of Dentists* 81.3: 14

'health research', including the study of any intervention that aims to change health-related behaviour on both individual and institutional levels.[18] This more inclusive conception clearly and significantly leaves room for the gauging of the proper amount of evidence for public health interventions.

A starting point for this type of assessment is the recognition of the fact that all health research – not only on biomedical interventions – imposes risks on research subjects, while the projected aim is to gather more knowledge in the interest of science or society.[19] A central tenet of research ethics therefore is that health research either has to plausibly benefit the research subject, or the societal benefit needs to be very large. In the new CIOMS guidelines, the latter is explicitly recognized in terms of the "social value" that may be attained by an intervention.[20] Furthermore, considerations of promoting trust towards health professionals and the complexity of the ethical issues involved provide arguments to treat health research with a certain amount of caution.[21] To this, we may add the precautionary considerations related in the preceding section: while a public health threat may be major and acute, any intervention meant to mitigate or prevent it may instead make it worse, or produce structural side effects that undermine other types of social goods. Therefore, the CIOMS frame is helpful to understand the question of evidence in public health interventions, such as the interventions aimed at fighting ABR.[22] To establish whether the evidence is sufficient, we have to chart the types of harm and uncertainty for various interventions in order to determine whether the expected (social) value of the intervention outweighs the value of postponing the use of a new intervention to collect more solid information about it.

This challenge is well illustrated by debates over suggested interventions in public health emergencies, such as Ebola.[23] When, in 2014, the West African Ebola epidemic was finally recognized as a global threat, it was suggested to prevent

---

[18] Council for International Organizations of Medical Sciences (CIOMS) (2016). International Ethical Guidelines for Health-Related Research Involving Humans. Geneva, Switzerland: Council for International Organizations of Medical Sciences. http://www.cioms.ch (accessed July 28, 2017). Munthe, C., Nijsingh, N., de Fine Licht, K., & Joakim Larsson, D. G. (2019). Health-related Research Ethics and Social Value: Antibiotic Resistance Intervention Research and Pragmatic Risks. Bioethics, 33(3), 335–342.

[19] Wilson, James, and David Hunter (2010). "Research exceptionalism." *American Journal of Bioethics* 10.8: 45–54.

[20] CIOMS (2016).

[21] Wilson and Hunter (2010).

[22] Attena, Francesco (2014). "Complexity and indeterminism of evidence-based public health: an analytical framework." *Medicine, Health Care and Philosophy* 17.3: 459–465.

[23] National Academies of Sciences, Engineering, and Medicine (2017). *Integrating Clinical Research into Epidemic Response: The Ebola Experience*. National Academies Press. An even more recent example is the Zika epidemic. See Edwards, Sarah JL (2016). "The precautionary paradox and Zika." *Research Ethics*: 178–181.

and Glenza, J. "Zika virus: Floridians fear 'Pandora's box' of genetically altered mosquitos." *The Guardian*, August 14, 2016: https://www.theguardian.com/us- news/2016/aug/14/florida-keys-zika-virus-genetically-modified-mosquitoes (accessed July 25, 2017).

further harm by 'fast tracking' new vaccines and experimental drugs, thus relaxing the demands of evidence required to introduce new medication.[24] This suggestion was countered by public health officials, who argued that the epidemic should rather be controlled by means of proven public health policies, such as proper hygiene, surveillance and quarantine.[25] Another issue that was debated was whether randomized clinical trials could be justified in the context of an epidemic and the extent to which genuine equipoise could be presumed. In part, the answers to these questions depend on the relative risk to which the affected communities were exposed, in another part it depends on how we assess the gravity of uncertainties underlying the assessment of these risks and how we value the importance of acting on good evidence in view of those uncertainties. While the question on the evidence of interventions to counter ABR is similar to such debates, the issue of ABR also raises a new set of worries and topics for discussion. Specifically, whereas the Ebola crisis was unexpected and presented an acute emergency, ABR is – for now – slowly emerging, albeit foreseen, but nevertheless posing a major and growing public health threat. Already a substantial amount of morbidity and mortality is attributed to ABR, but this number is likely to keep growing in a way well known to us.

Justifying Interventions

Since the causes are varied, the fight against ABR takes place in different arenas. In this section, we distinguish between various groups of interventions. The first set concerns the development of new types of (or alternatives for) antibiotics. Second, we consider interventions that target the access to antibiotics by individuals. Third, various interventions aim to establish a larger degree of surveillance. Last, we bring together various institutional measures to attack the environmental health side of the ABR problem, such as the use of antibiotics in animals, as well as emissions of antibiotics. In accordance with the broad notion of 'health research' introduced in the former section, these interventions span a wide array of different actions and policies. As a consequence, we will consider many different levels and types of intervention; both on the scale of an individual patient–doctor interaction, as well as on the level of macro-economic interventions, institutional regulation and global health treaties. Varied though these interventions may be, they all share the characteristic of aiming to help curbing – or otherwise fighting – ABR. To what extent it can be demonstrated that they are effective in that regard, and to what extent they pose risks of their own, determines whether they can be responsibly introduced.

Not all interventions in the fight against ABR are new. In fact, a number of important interventions intended to counter ABR belong to the classic public health

---

[24] Geisbert, Thomas W. (2015). "Emergency treatment for exposure to Ebola virus: the need to fast-track promising vaccines." Jama 313.12: 1221–1222.

[25] Rid, Annette, and Ezekiel J. Emanuel. (2014). "Ethical considerations of experimental interventions in the Ebola outbreak." *The Lancet* 384.9957: 1896–1899.

repertoire: screening, surveillance, quarantine, hygiene, and so on. Although they are not always uncontroversial, these interventions have been thoroughly tested and proven effective. Unfortunately, however, they will not suffice in addressing the problem of ABR.[26] New methods will need to be explored, which raises the question how to determine which intervention is preferable; which offers greater relative benefit, and which poses fewer relative risks? The answer to that question depends on the evidence available to assess the various interventions. We have no ambition here to be complete in listing the possible, but aim to illustrate and map some major complexities that arise when balancing the level of precaution against the price of precaution.

Biomedical Interventions

A fundamental problem in managing and fighting ABR is the lack of appropriate biomedical interventions. One aspect of this is *the lack of truly new antibiotics*. Although there is some progress in the development of novel antibiotics that affect Gram-positive bacteria (bacteria with a single outer cell wall),[27] innovation for Gram-negative bacteria that has reached the market has for decades consisted only in variations of the same.[28] In part, this can be attributed to the fact that developing new antibiotics is relatively unappealing from a business point of view. Therefore there is a widely recognized and urgent need to encourage academia and pharmaceutical companies to develop new antibiotics, and to facilitate their introduction.[29]

So-called *expedited programs* to this effect have been launched, for example by the US Food and Drug Administration (FDA).[30] Interventions included in such programs are priority review, accelerated approval, and fast track (which can be combined).[31] By promising a swifter, simplified and/or more relaxed process for licencing new therapies, such options both offer incentives to industry to invest in

---

[26] O'Neill, Jim (2014). Antimicrobial resistance: tackling a crisis for the health and wealth of nations. Review on antimicrobial resistance.

[27] Wright, Gerard. (2015). "Antibiotics: An irresistible newcomer." *Nature* 517.7535: 442–444.

[28] See, e.g., University of Illinois at Urbana-Champaign. "Antibiotic breakthrough: How to overcome gram-negative bacterial defenses." *ScienceDaily*. www.sciencedaily.com/releases/2017/05/170510132012.htm (accessed July 6, 2017); WHO 2015.

[29] World Health Organization, WHO. *Global priority list of antibiotic-resistant bacteria to guide research, discovery, and development of new antibiotics*. Geneva: World Health Organization, 2017. Online access: http://www.who.int/medicines/publications/global-priority-list-antibiotic-resistant-bacteria/en (accessed July 28, 2017)

[30] U.S. Department of Health and Human Services. *Guidance for Industry. Expedited Programs for Serious Conditions – Drugs and Biologics*. Washington: USDHHS, 2014. Online access: https://www.fda.gov/downloads/drugs/.../ucm358301.pdf *(accessed July 7, 2017)*. See for a more elaborate discussion: Munthe, C., & Nijsingh, N. (2019). Cutting red tape to manage public health threats: An ethical dilemma of expediting antibiotic drug innovation. Bioethics, 33(7), 785–791.

[31] https://www.fda.gov/forpatients/approvals/fast/ucm20041766.htm (accessed July 28, 2017)

the development of new antibiotics, and speed up the introduction of successful fruits of such endeavours. Interventions of this sort appear attractive, considering the potential damage that lack of development and delay could cause, motivating a lower acceptable price of precaution than in the case a "normal" drug development context. At the same time, entirely new classes of antibiotics imply elevated uncertainties regarding effect and side effects, pointing to a need for *more* caution, and motivating a higher price of precaution. In addition, problems with regards to the control of prescription, use and transmission imply further uncertainties regarding the benefits of "expediting" new antibiotics. In particular, it creates a stark tension between the overall aim of ABR research and the needs of patients burdened by resistant infections. If a new compound is introduced in a setting where the mentioned problems have not been mastered, resistance, though inevitable, can be expected to develop faster. As a result, there is a relative public health benefit to delay the discovery and introduction of new antibiotics while addressing the problems of ensuring responsible use, and mitigating transmission of resistance. Still, earlier introduction may save lives and reduce morbidity of individuals. Therefore, it is less clear whether expedited programs for the introduction of new antibiotics should be at the top of the priority list. Unless they are combined with effective measures to control usage and transmission, they introduce graver uncertainties of both negative side effects for patients, and of having the overall aim of managing the ABR problem undermined. Below, we will comment on interventions to manage this complexity of the ABR challenge.

Another aspect of this challenge is that, if resources are concentrated to this effect, it may be possible to develop drugs to take in order to mitigate plasmid-mediated transmission of resistant bacteria from one patient to others. These could be taken by patients with resistant infections, but also patients who take antibiotics where this treatment may otherwise give rise to local resistance. This is a possible intervention that is still in a very early stage of exploration,[32] which means there will be a long and expensive path to any possible actual treatment. At the same time, there is an obvious risk that no such success awaits at the other end – creating a severe uncertainty with regard to the actual worth of incentive schemes aimed at effecting such focused research and development endeavours. In addition, any successful treatment of this sort will create an ethical challenge in terms of exposing patients to the risk of side effects of the treatment without any sort of potential somatic benefit for these same patients. If it is successful, it will have an important general primary preventive effect of great public health value in the face of the ABR problem. If the introduction of such a drug would be "expedited", this will at the same time increase the risk and uncertainty regarding negative side effects concentrated only to those people taking the drug. Weighing these stakes has to be a part of striking the balance between what the acceptable price of precaution is to be when comparing incentive schemes.

[32] See, e.g., Buckner, Michelle, Maria Laura Ciusa, and Laura JV Piddock. (2018). "Strategies to combat antimicrobial resistance: anti-plasmid and plasmid curing." *FEMS microbiology reviews.*

Controlling use and transmission is less essential regarding therapeutic interventions where resistance development is not an apparent threat. Phage therapy (the therapeutic use of viral strains to attack bacteria) might fall into that category.[33] The efficacy and safety of phage therapy has not been proven to the stage where it would fulfil current guidelines in Europe and the USA. However, it might be that these guidelines do not quite suffice in assessing the responsible introduction of phage therapy, e.g. since individually designed cocktails may be required for each patient, creating an impediment for designing controlled trials. Thus, phage therapy, or other innovative solutions that do not (as new antibiotic compounds) feed immediately into the ABR development problem, may be a better target for "expedited programs" from an ABR standpoint – at least while we lack effective means to control use and transmission. On the other hand, accepting the higher degree of uncertainty, means lowering the level of required precaution, which may harm patients severely if experimental treatments turn out to be unsuccessful.

A more general challenge posed by all types of expediting program interventions, is that they may inadvertently create incentives that give rise to negative dynamics regarding drug development. The basic problem is that any expedited program creates an incentive for industry to re-direct their research efforts in a way that shapes studies to be less stringent and clinically relevant than what they would otherwise have been. A well-known example of this is the acceptance of surrogate outcome variables (an essential part of accelerated approval interventions), which makes it economically attractive for companies to run studies measuring only these, meaning that there will be a structural dynamic change of clinical research efforts into paths with less potential or without demonstrating actual clinical value. Similarly, so-called compassionate use programs have recently come under fire for creating a structural incentive for industry to move more and more drug development out of the default review process, thus creating a generally decreasing level of safety and elevated uncertainty regarding effect. To be sure, expediting programs partly aim at having industry thus allocate their efforts and resources, however, if there is a structural negative dynamic on the general effectiveness of new drugs, this must be viewed as a relevant downside. For that reason, policy makers may want to consider other solutions to the issue of drug development, such as rewarding pharmaceutical companies for developing new antibiotics, for example with exclusivity extensions, buyouts and entry prizes.[34] Each of these interventions has the potential to offer incentives to the pharmaceutical companies, but also to pose risks to society

---

[33] De Vos, Daniel & Pirnay, Jean-Paul (2015). "Could viruses help resolve the worldwide antibiotic crisis?" *AMR Control*, 110.

[34] Seth Seabury Neeraj Sood (2017, May 18). Toward A New Model For Promoting The Development Of Antimicrobial Drugs. *Health Affairs Blog*: http://healthaffairs.org/blog/2017/05/18/toward-a-new-model-for-promoting-the-development-of-antimicrobial-drugs/(accessed July 28, 2017); Morel, Chantal M., and Elias Mossialos. "Stoking the antibiotic pipeline." *BMJ: British Medical Journal (Online)* 340. Jim O'Neill (2014) has also suggested a ´pay or play´ principle, where pharmaceutical companies are required to either contribute or pay a fine.

and individuals, for instance a risk of social backlash.[35] There are, of course, also large uncertainties regarding whether or not such actions would be money well spent.

Returning to our main question concerning the evidence required for justifying various interventions that aim to offer incentives to develop new medicine, we see that a trade-off has to be made not just between individual and public interest, but also between various levels of uncertainty, and risks of structural negative dynamic effects. If faster development of antibiotics comes at the price of faster emergence of ABR for those same drugs, this raises the question on how to appreciate the urgency of the matter. In particular, it demands that we weigh current ABR against possible future ABR and the likelihood of developing alternatives for which ABR development is not an issue. There is both a danger of being retrospectively overly restrictive in the use of antibiotics when an alternative to the current drugs is found, as well as a danger of complacency based on the false reliance on such an alternative. At the same time, we need to weigh into the balance the apparent but uncertain risk of incentive schemes being structurally counterproductive.

Prescription Practices

Since the individual use of antibiotics is an important driver of ABR, interventions aiming to control the distribution of antibiotic drugs to individual patients are an important part of ABR policy. The proposed interventions include mandating prescription policies (in those countries where this is not already the case), various limitations to the type of antibiotics that are made available and improved access where antibiotics are currently lacking.

It is a received wisdom that the prescription system is an effective way of controlling the use of drugs. At the same time, the effectiveness on the system may vary, depending on numerous factors. For instance, antibiotic prescription practices across European regions vary considerably, linked to varying levels of institutional corruption.[36] Such structural challenges can be assumed to multiply in countries where there is no system or culture of effective prescription for antibiotics. Given the widespread acceptance of the over-the-counter availability of antibiotics in such societies, not only among citizens, but also medical professionals, and sometimes policy makers, there is a recognised uncertainty as to the real impact of trying to create or toughen up such regulation.[37]

---

[35] Munthe et al. (2019).

[36] Rönnerstrand, Björn, and Victor Lapuente. (2017). "Corruption and use of antibiotics in regions of Europe." Health Policy 121.3: 250–256.

[37] Radyowijati, Aryanti, and Hilbrand Haak (2003). "Improving antibiotic use in low-income countries: an overview of evidence on determinants." *Social science & medicine* 57.4 (2003): 733–744. Dreser, Anahí, et al. (2012). "Regulation of antibiotic sales in Mexico: an analysis of printed media coverage and stakeholder participation." BMC public health 12.1: 1051.

We meet here with a type of uncertainty that is entirely about how societies may react to attempted institutional change.[38] Weighing into the mix economic, cultural and institutional factors of relevance, a more incremental change seems preferable. It provides opportunity to attend to the interests of various stakeholders, as well as taking the time for a society to adjust, in order to ease both the passing of regulation, and its effective implementation. However, that requires quite a bit of knowledge of such mechanics of overarching social change, and also uses time itself as a factor. This raises the question of how long is long enough to attempt establishing social change, and how much effort should be spent on securing the understanding of how to make such attempts work. Facing the ABR challenge, how high should the price of precaution due to delaying prescription regulative action be allowed to rise while attending to such uncertainties?

For countries where a reasonably effective prescription practice is in place, unless a patient is critically ill, the first choice of antibiotics is often not the latest, most potent formula (with still limited resistance problems). Therefore, antibiotics prescribed usually bring a greater risk that the treatment will not cure the infection due to resistance. At the same time, this practice serves to protect the future integrity of "last line antibiotics" by minimising their use and thereby inhibiting the evolutionary drive towards resistance to them. Most commentators describe the payoff of these interventions in terms of *public good*, whereas risks of implementing them are considered to be carried by single *individuals*.[39] However, matters are slightly more complex than that. First, although there is agreement that this intervention does delay resistance for broad-spectrum compounds, the magnitude of the effect is still uncertain. Second, since broad-spectrum antibiotics are more likely to drive resistance in the individual patient's own gut flora,[40] there is also a chance of individual benefit linked to prescription practice.

We thus face a complex trade-off situation, where individual risks of suffering untreated infections must be balanced against the uncertain prospect that patients are protected against being infected by resistant bacteria, at the same time as the question remains whether this mix of risk and uncertain benefit for some individuals can be justified by a social benefit of uncertain magnitude. This also raises the question how much effort should be spent on making sure that the right balance is struck, for example by straightening out some of the important uncertainties.

In any case, agreeing that such a practice is indeed justified does not end the problem. We must also ask what intervention would actually effectively address it.

---

[38] The risk of incentive schemes for drug creation to produce unintended negative dynamics via their effect on industry in the former section also belongs to this type.

[39] Littmann, Jasper, and A. M. Viens. (2015). "The ethical significance of antimicrobial resistance." *Public health ethics* 8.3: 209–224.

[40] This is phenomenon can be observed in urinary tract infections, for example. As the normal non-resistant invading bacteria of this flora are exterminated by the treatment, a very fertile living space is created for bacteria that are resistant against the drug used. Costelloe, Ceire, et al. (2010). "Effect of antibiotic prescribing in primary care on antimicrobial resistance in individual patients: systematic review and meta-analysis." Bmj 340: c2096.

One idea, of course, is to make professional prescription guidelines for doctors to use. However, this introduces the uncertainty that doctors may fail to apply them, e.g., due to patient pressure, economic counter-incentives, or the mere inertness of habit. To address that, there is the option of allowing professionals less choice, for example by requiring application to a higher instance and proof of due cause for having a prescription green lighted. Such an intervention could consist of several levels of requirements, and for some antibiotics regular doctors may be stripped of all prescription rights. At the same time, being able to leave professional discretion to doctors in individual cases also has its value, and the more of rigid restriction is built into an intervention, the bigger the risk that individuals are harmed due to lack of (timely) access to treatment. However, rigid regulatory interventions clearly avoid the uncertainty with regard to the overall aims of delaying resistance development, as well as avoiding harmful individual prescriptions. To make this trade-off, it would be of great value to know more about the social dynamics creating the uncertainty around the effectiveness of prescription interventions, as well as how these might be complemented by additional institutional changes to mitigate the pressure on doctors from patients, and to remove economic counter-incentives.[41] On the other hand, as we delay action, or apply overly cautious interventions with uncertain effectiveness while making sure what more exact variant would be best, the price of precaution is allowed to go up in terms present prescription practices being allowed to continue.

This precautionary challenge is further complicated by the fact that there is an instrumental value to fine-tune prescription interventions so that treatment of infection is optimized also under a restrictive prescription practice. The reason for this is that increased persistent infection can be expected to increase the future demand and consumption of antibiotics, thereby accelerating rather than mitigating resistance development in the long run.[42] Depending on what current prescription practices look like in specific societies, this may mean that an optimal prescription intervention should not only decrease prescription, but in some cases leave it as it is, and in yet other even *improve* the access to antibiotics. Considerations of fairness may add further reasons to a similar effect, and also the need of securing the legitimacy of any policy in this area. After all, of what interest is the issue of ABR to anyone who is barred from accessing appropriate antibiotics in the first place? This further complicates the uncertainty about what exact intervention would be most effective. But it also adds a basic source of uncertainty with regard to how the moral stakes should be balanced in a measure of effectiveness. A sound precautionary solution therefore needs to acknowledge the latter point when striking the balance between ensuring a desired level of precaution at an acceptable price of precaution, and allow both considerations of health promotion and fair distribution of the population health.

---

[41] As such changes may involve drastic reform to entire health care and health insurance systems, the knowledge required is quite advanced and complicated to collect.

[42] Daulaire, N., et al. (2015). "Universal access to effective antimicrobials: an essential feature of global collective action against antimicrobial resistance." *Journal of Law, Medicine & Ethics* 43.2.

Surveillance

The fight against ABR also requires enhanced possibilities of diagnosis and surveillance of resistant bacteria. Better diagnostic methods are in themselves unobjectionable as increased speed, precision and readiness in determining the cause of an infection limits the danger of squandering antibiotics. However, there will be trade-offs between increasing speed, increasing precision and financial costs and possibly the intrusiveness of the sample taking. Because of this, as well as the general uncertainties befalling any new measurement tool, there is once again a challenge to decide how much support for the reliability and validity of a new diagnostic tool has to be secured in order to start implementing it. The balance here, as before, includes assessing the value of more firm knowledge against the price of precaution in terms of delaying tools that may also offer opportunities for better surveillance in the face of the ABR threat. But it also includes the complications as more speedy introduction will tend to increase one or the other of well-known downsides to such interventions.

These complications become especially challenging as resistant infections or even carriership may often actualise restrictive communicable disease management measures, such as compulsory isolation, quarantine or mandatory life-style restrictions. The implied tension between individual interest and collective good is particularly salient when this involves asymptomatic carriers, who have nothing to benefit from being institutionalized.[43] The issue is further complicated when we consider the possibility of false positives, where patients are wrongly identified as carrying resistant bacteria. As in the former section, this also links to a risk of undermining the legitimacy of ABR policies. Thus, while speedy introduction of diagnostic methods certainly has its potential upsides, it will increase uncertainties of a sort that in other areas are often taken to undermine health surveillance programs.

Attempting to strike these several balances, we face the general problem of having the right idea concerning the moral stakes involved and a sound notion of what price of precaution to allow. In addition, increased complexities of how to assess the quality of available and attainable evidence for ambitious and complex public health interventions add another layer of uncertainty.[44]

[43] Weinstein, Robert A., Daniel J. Diekema, and Michael B. Edmond. (2007). "Look before you leap: active surveillance for multidrug-resistant organisms." Clinical Infectious Diseases 44.8: 1101–1107. Nijsingh, N., Juth, N., Munthe, C., "The Ethics of Screening", in: Quah, Stella R. International encyclopedia of public health. Academic Press, 2016. Nijsingh, N., Munthe, C., Lindblom, A., & Åhrén, C. (2020). Screening for multi-drug-resistant Gram-negative bacteria: what is effective and justifiable?. Monash bioethics review.

[44] Attena, (2014).

Environment and Animals

A wide variety of ABR interventions relate to attempts to curb the emission of antibiotics in the environment[45] and their use in animals. We have grouped these together because of the potential risks of the interventions, which seem mostly economical. For example, attempts to enhance transparency of pharmaceutical companies[46]or banning of the use of antibiotics as a growth enhancer,[47] or taxing consumer products emanating from ABR driving practices, such as meat production,[48] do not have direct health risks for humans. Compared to the possible economic damage of such interventions, the health risks of ABR may seem to clearly win out. However, there is still much uncertainty concerning the role of non-human use and pollution in the establishing of ABR and economic cost of interventions carry their own set of secondary risks and uncertainties, which might be substantial indeed as the incurred costs become more significant.

One obvious uncertainty regards the effectiveness of systems of surveillance and control of emission rates in production or compound use in farming. These will include uncertainties and imprecisions of technical methods, but even more institutional uncertainties of the sort we have already discussed related to prescription and surveillance interventions. As already observed, straightening these uncertainties out includes coming to grips with very complex social circumstances, and may require quite a lot of time and resources.

On top of this, macro-economic ABR interventions targeting environmental emission may have adverse effects in themselves, both socially and economically, for instance, by discouraging pharmaceutical business and thereby restricting access to drugs generally. Consequently, we may legitimately ask which interventions are necessary, or reasonable, and which are disproportional, given the uncertain effects of current practices. Should, for instance, pharmaceutical companies be required to monitor and make sure antibiotics emission from manufacturing are very low?[49] Or should regulation rather target the pricing of products, adding tax or extra cost in the procurement of drugs by public national health services? Or should some other

---

[45] Pruden, Amy, et al. "Management options for reducing the release of antibiotics and antibiotic resistance genes to the environment." *Environmental health perspectives* 121.8 (2013): 878.

[46] Larsson, DG Joakim, and Jerker Fick. "Transparency throughout the production chain—a way to reduce pollution from the manufacturing of pharmaceuticals?." *Regulatory Toxicology and Pharmacology* 53.3 (2009): 161–163. Nijsingh, N., Munthe, C., & Larsson, D. J. (2019). Managing pollution from antibiotics manufacturing: charting actors, incentives and disincentives. Environmental Health, 18(1), 95.

[47] Laxminarayan, Ramanan, Thomas Van Boeckel, and Aude Teillant. (2015). "The economic costs of withdrawing antimicrobial growth promoters from the livestock sector.".

[48] Giubilini, Alberto, et al. (2017). "Taxing Meat: Taking Responsibility for One's Contribution to Antibiotic Resistance." *Journal of Agricultural and Environmental Ethics* 30.2: 179–198.

[49] Bengtsson-Palme, Johan, and DG Joakim Larsson. (2016). "Concentrations of antibiotics predicted to select for resistant bacteria: Proposed limits for environmental regulation." *Environment International* 86: 140–149.

institutional intervention to similar effect be chosen, for example having high emissions in production reduce the calculated health benefit in the context of health technology assessment? In all these cases, should the link between detected emission rates and such incentives be proportionally or more rigidly designed? If the former, according to what formula or proportionality, if the latter, on what grounds should thresholds be set? And what institutional arrangement would be effective to have whatever intervention is chosen to be effectively implemented? Similar questions appear with regard to interventions aimed at creating incentives to reduce the use of antibiotics in farming.[50]

All of this makes for a considerable difficulty in assessing the proper balancing of the level of precaution and its acceptable price. Surely, the urgency of mitigating major environmental practices that fuel antibiotic resistance development is a priority. However, to find the right way of doing this requires quite a bit of very complex knowledge, and behind this need lurks the very real risk that a more speedy introduction of interventions is not only sub-optimal, but actually makes the problem worse. For instance, implementing any of the regulative interventions mentioned may mainly have the effect of having pharmaceutical and food production relocating to areas where the regulative situation is even worse. Or secondary effects, e.g., in the form of drastically increased food prices may both undermine the legitimacy of ABR policies and create a public health threat of its own. On the other hand, it is well known that it takes considerable time to have large-scale operations such as drug production and farming change their longstanding ways, and in the light of that, applying interventions to address the environmental side of the ABR challenge is paramount.

Discussion

We have assessed interventions with regard to how much and what kind of evidence is needed when evaluating and implementing interventions in response to antibiotic resistance, a public health threat of immense proportions. The notion of responsible precautionary decision-making provides a basic and strong reason to act in response to this threat. However, determining *what* response to go for introduces complex problems of balancing what level of precaution to aim for and what price of precaution to pay, actualising much more difficult ethical challenges than what is often acknowledged.

We end this exploration by briefly addressing two issues that emerge when we consider the evidence for interventions that aim to fight antibiotic resistance, leading into a final broad suggestion for future analyses to build on.

[50] Silley, Peter, and Bernd Stephan. (2017). "Prudent use and regulatory guidelines for veterinary antibiotics—politics or science?." *Journal of applied microbiology* 123.6: 1373–1380.

First, there is the sheer size of the possible consequences of increased ABR. For example, there is a real question whether standards of treatment and diagnosis in research ethics and clinical ethics may need revision in light of a public health threat as significant to global wellbeing as ABR. Although one should be wary to discard too easily the frameworks that have proven to be of value throughout the years, the possible disruptive effects of ABR raise the issue to what extent these standards can be maintained, given the range of difficult choices we might face. At the same time, we have seen that many of the uncertainties posed by ABR interventions are not so much about having risks of undesirable side effects as such are typically conceived of when evaluating pharmaceuticals. Rather, the important uncertainties are about risks of outright counterproductivity due to social psychological and institutional dynamics, where apparently promising attempts to counter ABR may instead lure us into political, economic or psychological dead ends from which we are unable to get out. Social processes are typically slow, variably inert and intractable, which means also that they may be very difficult to reverse, and that doing so may require a lot of time. Given that interventions on all of the mentioned levels are probably necessary to reduce the risk of emerging resistance and that they are to a large extent interrelated, the standards of evidence should be set from an integrated, One Health perspective.

This connects to the general observation that methods in response to ABR have to intervene on a variety of different levels, from the everyday practice of physicians to those affecting global structures. Interventions worthy of consideration therefore involve a myriad of different types and degrees of uncertainty and risks, which are also unevenly distributed across people, societies and time. Assessment of the evidence thus needs to consider a multi-layered mosaic of uncertainties and ethical dilemmas regarding the short- and long-term trade-off between individual interests and public health aims. This regards especially the issue of how much and what evidence to collect regarding the effectiveness of interventions, and their potential long-term legitimacy.

These considerations may drive one to despair whether a responsible, measured approach to the issues at play here is at all feasible. One way of moving forward in the light of these considerations is to acknowledge that there are good – moral *and* precautionary – reasons to cut the Gordian knot: just as there is a question of how much to amass and ponder evidence and the proper resolution of ethical dilemmas, we must not get stuck forever in the precautionary conundrum. Moving along such a path, one primary consideration is then to assess the relative importance of avoiding harm and risk of harm that result from otherwise apparently effective intervention packages, while avoiding the pull of the enormity of the ABR challenge to lure us into policy deadlocks. In doing so, the complexity and close connections of the various risks offer strong grounds for putting the reversibility of potential adverse consequences at centre stage. Related to debates on the ethics of precaution, this links to different proposals on how to limit the scope of a precautionary principle, e.g., in terms of *de minimis* risk, and, more specifically, to the importance of avoiding irreversible negative outcomes. This is not to say that this is a generally plausible solution for all precautionary decision-making, but the peculiar complex challenges of assessing evidence for ABR interventions seem to add reasons for the fittingness of an approach that prioritises reversibility.[51]

[51] This research was supported by the UGOT Challenges Initiative at the University of Gothenburg; and by the Swedish Research Coucil, VR, contract no. 2014–40, for the Lund-Gothenburg Responsibility Project.

11

Global Governance of Anti-microbial Resistance: A Legal and Regulatory Toolkit

Calvin W. L. Ho and Tsung-Ling Lee

Abstract Recognizing that antimicrobial resistance (AMR) poses a serious threat to global public health, the World Health Organization (WHO) has adopted a Global Action Plan (GAP) at the May 2015 World Health Assembly. Underscoring that systematic misuse and overuse of drugs in human medicine and food production is a global public health concern, the GAP-AMR urges concerted efforts across governments and private sectors, including pharmaceutical industry, medical professionals, agricultural industry, among others. The GAP has a threefold aim: (1) to ensure a continuous use of effective and safe medicines for treatment and prevention of infectious diseases; (2) to encourage a responsible use of medicines; and (3) to engage countries to develop their national actions on AMR in keeping with the recommendations. While the GAP is a necessary step to enable multilateral actions, it must be supported by effective governance in order to realize the proposed aims.

This chapter has a threefold purpose: (1) To identify regulatory principles embedded in key WHO documents relating to AMR and the GAP-AMR; (2) To consider the legal and regulatory actions or interventions that countries could use to strengthen their regulatory lever for AMR containment; and (3) To highlight the crucial role of the regulatory lever in enabling other levers under a whole-of-system approach. Effective AMR containment requires a clearer understanding of how the regulatory lever could be implemented or enabled within health systems, as well as how it underscores and interacts with other levers within a whole-of-system approach.

C. W. L. Ho (✉)
Faculty of Law, The University of Hong Kong, Hong Kong S.A.R., People's Republic of China

Centre for Medical Ethics and Law, Li Ka Shing School of Medicine and Faculty of Law, The University of Hong Kong, Hong Kong S.A.R., People's Republic of China
e-mail: cwlho@hku.hk

T.-L. Lee
Taipei Medical University, Taipei, Taiwan

Shuang-Ho Hospital, New Taipei City, Taiwan
e-mail: tl265@georgetown.edu

Keywords Global action plan · Governance · Regulation · Law/legal · Collective action · Stewardship

Introduction

Antimicrobial resistance (AMR) is widely recognized as a public health threat, responsible for 700,000 deaths worldwide. If the spread of antimicrobial resistance is left unaddressed, it could lead to 10 million additional annual deaths by 2050, according to an estimation by the World Bank. Facilitated by inappropriate uses of medicines to control the spread of infection for human and animal health, antimicrobial resistance also poses long term threat to human development. The United Nations (UN) Secretary-General Ban Ki-Moon describes AMR as a "fundamental threat" to human development at a high-level UN meeting on drug-resistant bacteria (United Nations News Centre 2016). Likewise, recognizing the gravity of antimicrobial resistance on global health, the then Director-General for the World Health Organization (WHO) Margaret Chan characterizes the rise of AMR as a "slow-motion tsunami" (Leatherby 2017). Without an effective global containment strategy, the World Bank warns, the economic impact of AMR makes it unlikely for the world to reach the sustainable development goals set for 2030 (World Bank 2017).

Scientists have long known that microbes can become resistant to medicine. Alexander Fleming, the Nobel laureate for the discovery of penicillin, cautioned the world in his 1945 Nobel acceptance speech of the impending public health crisis (Fleming 1945, at p. 93): "… there is the danger that the ignorant man may easily under dose himself and by exposing his microbes to non-lethal quantities of the drug make them resistant." Since the 1950s the WHO has identified AMR as a global threat, but little progress has been made in improving access to antimicrobials and maintaining their appropriate consumption and effectiveness. Likewise, limited innovation in antimicrobials further compounds the challenge. For these reasons, a broad range of microorganisms have become more resistant to antimicrobials in all parts of the world. An emerging concern is AMR for diseases which affect low and middle income countries (LMICs) disproportionately, such as tuberculosis (TB), malaria and HIV (See Chaps. 2–4). Furthermore, with extensively drug-resistant to tuberculosis now identified in 105 countries, it further raises concerns of a future TB epidemic where limited treatment options are available.

Even though the direct consequences of AMR on human health were beginning to be scientifically well-understood several decades ago, international efforts to address this problem did not begin till the late 1990s and 2000s. The WHO played a key role in catalysing international actions on the issue. It convened a series of consultative groups and expert workshop to assess, evaluate, and develop a series of recommendation for effective containment interventions to garner international attention. This work culminated in the report *WHO Global Strategy for Containment of Antimicrobial Resistance* (World Health Organization 2001). Since this strategy was published, AMR has been discussed at several World Health Assembly meetings, resulting in the adoption of several resolutions such as WHA60.16 concerning the rational use of medicine and WHA62.15 on prevention and control of multidrug-resistant tuberculosis and extensively drug-resistant tuberculosis. At the 2015 World Health Assembly, member states endorsed a *Global Action Plan on Antimicrobial Resistance* (GAP-AMR; World Health Organization 2015a) – which calls for an effective One Health approach – and which was later endorsed through resolutions by the Food and Agriculture Organization of the United Nations (FAO) and World Organisation for Animal Health (OIE). In the same year, AMR was recognized as a threat to the world's sustainability and human development at the UN level. In a landmark UN resolution guiding the global development plan for the next 15 years entitled *Transforming our world: the 2030 Agenda for Sustainable Development* (United Nations 2015), AMR is mentioned but not explicitly set out as a Sustainable Development Goals (SDGs) target. Most recently, the G20 summit reaffirmed the commitment to combat antimicrobial resistance (G20 Leaders' Declaration 2017).

These commitments, both within and outside of the high-level political setting of UN organs, underscore the growing political interest in AMR. Two distinct but interrelated factors explain the recent high-level political attention. First, national governments have a strong self-interest in mitigating the negative impacts of AMR on public health: the estimated economic cost for failing to address the issue would be £66 trillion in lost productivity to the global economy (Public Health England 2015). Second, AMR transcends national borders and exposes a global vulnerability which necessitates collective action at the international level. The shared vulnerability underpinning AMR was recently acknowledged by Tedros Adhanom, the WHO Director-General, in his address to the G20 summit. Urging the world to act, he underscored the interdependence of the world, noting "… vulnerability for one is vulnerability for all of us" (World Health Organization 2017a). German Chancellor Angela Merkel echoed this concern, depicting AMR as akin to a global health security issue of global collective responsibility (Scheuber 2017).

This chapter has a threefold purpose: (1) To identify regulatory principles embedded in key WHO documents relating to AMR and the GAP-AMR; (2) To consider the legal and regulatory actions or interventions that countries could use to strengthen their regulatory lever for AMR containment; and (3) To highlight the crucial role of the regulatory lever in enabling other levers under a whole-of-system approach. In the section that follows, we consider how the WHO and other international bodies have systematically framed this global health issue as a collective action problem; initially by setting out the WHO GAP-AMR. But subsequently, it was quickly recognised that a global plan would not be self-enabling and therefore a global framework has since been proposed by the UN to facilitate implementation by all member states. We set out what we consider to be the core principles that are embedded in the GAP-AMR and the global framework built around it. We then consider the regulatory lever that member states need to establish and apply in order for these principles to effect change at the national level.

The WHO and AMR

Collective Action Problem

Ilona Kickbusch and David Gleicher (World Health Organization 2012a, b) define global health as health issues which transcend national boundaries and governments and call for actions on the global forces and global flows that determine the health of people. As microbes are capable of penetrating national borders, national efforts are contingent upon, and vulnerable to external actions and forces. It is widely recognised that a collective response is necessary to mitigate the negative consequences of AMR. As no country is capable of addressing the issue without some degree of mutual reliance on others to mount an effective response against AMR, the interdependency makes AMR containment a collective action problem.

Some scholars go further and argue that the containment of AMR is a public good: the benefits from effective containment are enjoyed by all and there is no rivalry in consumption (Smith and Coast 2002). If this is correct, it could present a free rider problem: individual states lack incentive to take the necessary actions and instead, rely on others to act. Arguably, the free rider problem can be addressed through international law (Wernli et al. 2011; Review on Antimicrobial Resistance 2014). Steven Hoffman and Asha Behdinan (2016), Reinl (2016), Susan Rogers Van Katwyk et al. (2016), Christine Årdal et al. (2016), and Asha Behdinan et al. (2015), for instance, argue that countries can be encouraged to act if international law embeds incentives. While many international institutions are involved in addressing the threat posed by AMR, as a starting point, we focus the discussion on the WHO, particularly for its instrumental role in developing the GAP-AMR.

Global Action Plan

Recognizing that systematic misuse and overuse of antimicrobial drugs in human medicine and food production puts every nation at risk, the overarching goal of the GAP-AMR is thus to ensure that the world is able to "treat and prevent infectious diseases with effective and safe medicines that are quality-assured, used in a responsible way, and accessible to all who need them" (World Health Organization 2015a, b, at p. 8). To achieve this goal, the GAP-AMR requires concurrent actions at the national and international levels. While the GAP-AMR is not technically binding, it seeks to harmonise practices across countries while affording regulatory flexibility. To assure policy coherence at the national and international levels, the GAP-AMR provides five objectives to guide and align national and international policy actions: (1) to improve awareness and understanding of AMR through effective communication, education and training; (2) to strengthen the knowledge and evidence base through surveillance and research; (3) to reduce the incidence of infection through effective sanitation, hygiene and infection prevention measures; (4) to optimize the use of antimicrobial medicines in human and animal health; and (5) to develop the economic case for sustainable investment that takes account of the needs of all countries, and increases investment in new medicines, diagnostic tools, vaccines and other interventions. Member states are urged to have national action plans that are aligned with the GAP-AMR within 2 years of the endorsement of the action plan by the World Health Assembly.

Moreover, because excessive human and animal use of antibiotics in multiple settings will have health, economic and security implications beyond national borders, the GAP-AMR embraces a *One Health* approach towards AMR. Defined as a collaborative, multi-sectoral and trans-disciplinary, the *One Health* approach recognizes interconnection between people, animals, plants and the shared environment. This approach calls for sectorial coordination involving human and veterinary medicine, agriculture, finance, environment, and consumers to optimal health outcomes. At the level of international health, horizontal coordination of different UN agencies occurs through the WHO. As the specialized public health agency within the UN agency, the WHO is charged with organizing international responses to shared health challenges, and this responsibility includes acting as "the directing and coordinating authority on international health work" (World Health Organization n. d.). The WHO works with the Strategic and Technical Advisory Group on AMR at the FAO and OIE to develop a framework for monitoring and evaluation of member states' national action plans. Likewise, the FAO, OIE and World Bank are encouraged to put in place and implement action plans in their respective fields. Notably, the regulatory functions bestowed on the WHO are broader in scope than any other international agency in the UN orbit.

As of 2017, more than one third of WHO member states have completed their national action plans on AMR, and a further 62 are in the process of doing so. These national action plans provide a basis for an assessment of the resource needs at national and international levels. The WHO is tasked with publishing biennial progress report on countries' progress in implementing their national action plans. The progress report will also include an assessment of progress made by the FAO, OIE and WHO.

Limitations of the Global Action Plan

To be sure, the GAP-AMR provides a good starting point, but the plan lacks concrete goals to compel action. Moreover, the WHO alone cannot be expected to solve the global AMR crisis. For instance, preserving antimicrobial medicines will require a global agreement as to what constitutes 'appropriate use'. Likewise, new financing mechanisms will be needed to incentivise global innovation in antimicrobial medicines. Thus, in the same resolution that endorsed the global action plan, the World Health Assembly (2015a, b) requested the Director-General to develop a global development and stewardship framework to support GAP-AMR in combating AMR. Specifically, the Health Assembly requires the Director-General to (World Health Assembly 2015a, b, Request 7):

> develop, in consultation with Member States and relevant partners, options for establishing a global development and stewardship framework to support the development, control, distribution and appropriate use of new antimicrobial medicines, diagnostic tools, vaccines and other interventions, while preserving existing antimicrobial medicines, and promoting affordable access to existing and new antimicrobial medicines and diagnostic tools, taking into account the needs of all countries, and in line with the global action plan on antimicrobial resistance.

The global framework will build on the GAP-AMR, but with specific focuses on preservation of antimicrobial medicines and development of new antimicrobial medicines, diagnostic tools, vaccines and other interventions. According to a report issued by the FAO, OIE and WHO (Food and Agriculture Organization 2017, at p. 4), a global development and stewardship framework would have a threefold goal:

1. Stewardship: Preserving antimicrobial medicines through a stewardship framework covering control, distribution and appropriate use;
2. Research & Development: Developing of new health technologies for preventing and controlling antimicrobial resistance; and
3. Access: Promoting affordable access to existing and new antimicrobial medicines and diagnostic tools.

This framework further encapsulates key principles that have been expounded in earlier initiatives of the WHO. For the purposes of this chapter, we highlight three principles that are of especial pertinence to laws and regulations on pharmaceuticals, which are discussed in the section that follows (for a broader ethical discussion on AMR, see Haire, Chap. 3, this volume; Cheah et al., Chap. 4, this volume). Not necessarily in order of priority, these principles are:

1. Rational and responsible use of antimicrobials

At a practical level, the WHO defines rational use of medicines as patients receiving medications appropriate to their clinical needs, in doses that meet their own individual requirements, for an adequate period of time, and at the lowest cost to them and their community (World Health Organization 1985). This definition extends to the use of antimicrobials, where for instance, irrational use occurs when patients are prescribed and/or take antibiotics (intended to treat bacterial infection) when in fact they have a viral infection. As a matter of public policy, responsible use of antimicrobials is set out as a governing principle that should underpin national governments' efforts to curb AMR. This principle requires governments to ensure that existing activities, capabilities and resources of health system are aligned to ensure patients receive the right dosage of antimicrobials at the right time, use them appropriately and benefit from the usage (World Health Organization 2012a, b).

2. Equitable access to, and appropriate use of, existing and new antimicrobial medicines.

The GAP-AMR recognizes that all countries should have a national action plan on antimicrobial resistance that includes an assessment of resource needs. Moreover, recognizing the need to optimise the use of antimicrobial medicines in human and animal health, the WHO has updated its model list of essential medicine which categories antibiotics into three groups: access, watch and reserve. The access group include antibiotics (considered to have low resistance potential) recommended as first or second choice treatment options for common infections. This group of antibiotics should be widely available at an affordable cost and of assured quality. The watch group of antibiotics are those generally considered as to have higher resistance potential but are recommended as for first or second choice treatment for limited number of indicators. The reserve group consists of 'last-resort' options, or tailored to highly specific patients and setting, and when other alternatives have already failed. International efforts are required in monitoring, reporting the uses of reserve antibiotics to preserve their effectiveness (World Health Organization 2017b, c).

3. Transparency: Data Sharing, Collection and Evaluation

Data sharing, collection and evaluation have been emphasised in order to promote transparency and collaboration. A report by the WHO Secretariat on antimicrobial resistance sets these responsibilities out concisely as (World Health Organization 2015a, at p. 11): "Publishing biennial progress reports, including an assessment of countries and organizations that have plans in place, their progress in implementation, and the effectiveness of action at regional and global levels; and including an assessment of progress made by the FAO, OIE and WHO in implementing actions undertaken within the organizations' tripartite collaboration will also be included in these reports."

Significantly, the call for a global development and stewardship framework was later reiterated at a high-level meeting on antimicrobial resistance at the UN level in 2016 (United Nations 2016). It was the only fourth time that the UN General Assembly convened a high-level meeting on a health issue. Previous meetings – HIV/AIDS, Ebola and non-communicable diseases – catalysed and mobilized political actions at the international level. The UN Political Declaration on antimicrobial resistance was adopted by all 193 member states, signalling a global commitment to combat antimicrobial resistance.

In the discussion so far, we have considered the framing of AMR as a collective action problem the WHO and other international organisations. We have also briefly set out how the GAP-AMR and an enabling global framework have been constructed in response to this problem. More importantly, we have attempted to identify key principles that are embedded in the GAP-AMR, and in respect of which the global framework seeks to give expression to. For ease of reference, we refer to them generally as regulatory principles, because member states need to incorporate them – through laws and regulations – within their health systems. These laws and regulations collectively constitute a regulatory lever that will, at a basic level, enable member states to design, implement and manage policies (particularly pharmaceutical oriented ones) toward responsible use and good stewardship of antimicrobials. These laws and regulations are considered in the next section of the chapter. We then explain why a sound regulatory lever within a whole-of-system approach is critical to enable other levers (financial and information ones in particular) to operate effectively in meeting global AMR objectives.

Regulatory Leverage for Responsible Use and Good Stewardship of Antimicrobials

The prevalence of AMR is heavily influenced by the way that antimicrobials are consumed. It is now well established that overuse and underuse of antibiotics can lead to resistance (Jamrozik and Selgelid, Chap. 1, this volume). Even so, improper or imprudent use of antibiotics is deeply entrenched within health systems. In order for all member states of the WHO to meet their moral and political commitments set out under the GAP-AMR, it is critical for health systems to be strengthened on all fronts. Clearly the challenge of AMR is a complex one because it is influenced by many different factors and conditions. At the level of health systems, the relational dynamics between prescribers (or suppliers) of antibiotics and patients (or consumers), financial incentives, systemic commitments and characteristics, and the regulatory environment, are arguably the key contributors to AMR. For the purposes of this chapter, we focus on the role of regulation (broadly applied to refer to both legislative and regulatory actions) and examine how it could be used to support the containment of AMR. Many countries do not have a substantially clear and systematic legal and regulatory framework that is specifically directed at AMR (for example, Singh 2017). At a fundamental level, a clear regulatory position on responsible antimicrobial use that simultaneously prioritises effective antimicrobial stewardship is a pre-requisite to a coordinated response in policy decisions and actions across different domains within a health system. In addition, a variety of regulatory interventions should be considered to enable, as well as promote, the use of structural (delivery arrangement), information and financial levers to encourage appropriate use and stewardship of antimicrobials. It is further important for the regulatory environment to be sufficiently open in allowing a combination of top-down and bottom-up actions within a whole-of-system approach.

Policy discussions on effective stewardship of pharmaceuticals in health systems as a response to the problem of AMR predate the GAP-AMR. In a WHO report (Bigdeli et al. 2014) published ahead of the 2015 World Health Assembly, four main policy objectives with respect to medicines (and antimicrobials) in health systems have been identified as: (1) widely available high-quality medicinal products; (2) equitable access; (3) appropriate and safe use; and (4) affordability. Different policy actions and conditions are matched to each of the four policy objectives in the following manner (Bigdeli et al. 2014, at p. 45):

1. Ensuring availability of quality generic and innovative products:
    - Monitoring product quality;
    - Prequalifying supplies and products;

- Negotiating prices, quality, volume, and supply-chain security;
- Promoting fair competition;
- Engaging in risk sharing agreements;
- Establishing patient access programmes;

2. Improving Equitable Access:
   - Understanding utilization profiles;
   - Assessing of care seeking behaviour and barriers to care;
   - Expanding provider networks;
   - Targeting policies and programmes to improve access for vulnerable populations;
3. Encouraging Appropriate Use:
   - Implementing and updating standard treatment guidelines;
   - Matching essential medicines and reimbursement lists to standard treatment guidelines;
   - Assessing provider performance;
   - Managing care comprehensively;
   - Implementing and monitoring policies to encourage clinically appropriate and cost-effective use;
4. Keeping cost affordable:
   - Monitoring routine medicines expenditures by therapeutic area;
   - Evaluating health technologies and budget impact;
   - Assessing household medicines expenditure;
   - Implementing and monitoring policies and programmes to reduce waste and inappropriate use.

Not surprisingly, these policy objectives are closely aligned with what we have identified to be regulatory principles that underscore the GAP-AMR. For instance, rational and responsible use, equitable access and transparency are all necessary conditions to ensure the availability of quality antimicrobials within a health system. However, these policy objectives and their attending actions and conditions inevitably compete in many ways. Price pressures could limit investment in governance infrastructure, where such limitations are typically manifested in weak regulatory capacity, information imbalance, lack of coordination among different stakeholders and perverse incentives whereby irresponsible use is directly supported by direct financial gain. Over time, these practices not only strain health systems by increasing needless consumption, cost and inefficiencies, but also accentuate the global threat of AMR. Within the paradigm of value-based practice, the problem of AMR highlights the urgent need to shift current low-value practices to high-value ones (Porter 2010; Elshaug et al. 2017). A low-value practice is an intervention where evidence suggests that it confers no or very little benefit (to a patient for instance). It also depicts any practice where risk of harm exceeds probable benefit, or where added costs of the intervention do not provide proportional added benefits.

In contrast, a high-value practice is one where evidence suggests it confers benefit on the intervention subject, or probability of benefit exceeds probable harm, or where the added costs of the intervention provide proportional added benefits relative to alternatives. For instance, overprescribing that is incentivised, among other factors, by increased revenue for healthcare providers through greater pharmaceutical sales is a low-value practice that continues to be sustained in many health systems.

While it is beyond the scope of this chapter to address comprehensively the value implications of inappropriate use and poor stewardship of antimicrobials, our intent is to make explicit an implicit understanding that responding to the AMR challenge could be closely linked to addressing many on-going concerns relating to quality of care (World Health Organization 2016). The role and impact of regulation on quality of care have been a longstanding concern among a variety of scholars in different quarters. With limited exception however (notably in the work on refining the working definitions for substandard and falsified medical products (World Health Organization 2017c)), there has not been as much focus on the regulatory lever within health systems on containment of AMR as compared to the financial lever, for example. We hope to address this deficiency by proposing different tools and conditions that could make-up or compose the regulatory lever in relation to each of the four policy objectives identified by the WHO, as well as propose what we consider to be a sufficient open and responsive regulatory environment that could constructively resolve tensions by focusing on higher-value practice when these objectives come into conflict.

Ensuring Quality

A sufficiently robust and up-to-date legal and regulatory framework is necessary to control the quality, safety and efficacy of pharmaceuticals, including antimicrobials. Substandard or degraded antimicrobials, where dosage may be lower or less effective, contribute to therapeutic failure and could thereby encourage the development of drug-resistant strain of pathogens. Similarly, counterfeit antimicrobials could have an adverse effect if the active ingredients include other types of antibiotics (and/or other drugs). In order for such a legal and regulatory framework to be robust, regulatory actions must include accreditation, audit and inspection for the purposes of controlling quality and assessing the safety and efficacy of antimicrobials. For instance, health systems that manufacture antimicrobials must have a legal and regulatory framework to ensure that good manufacturing standards and practices are adhered to. It is not enough to only specify these requirements, but it is just as important for regulatory mechanisms to be in place that can effectively detect deficiencies or deviations from prescribed standards and practices.

Appropriate laws and regulations are also needed to legitimise, implement and sustain policies and programmes that are directed at rational and appropriate antimicrobial use. These policies and programmes generally relate to disease surveillance and management, and standard treatment guidelines. More recently, various measures have been introduced to incentivise the use of high value care through pay-for-performance programmes. These programmes reward healthcare providers for achieving quality, efficiency and "value" by increasing accessibility and appropriate use of drugs that are of proven efficacy. However, evidence of the effectiveness of such programmes are mixed in high-income countries and extremely limited in LMICs. From a regulatory standpoint, pay-for-performance programmes are not self-enabling everywhere but are likewise dependent on a supportive regulatory environment. Broadly speaking, appropriate legal or regulatory principles should be in place to ensure fair bargain, safety and (where appropriate) fair compensation, monitoring and data sharing.

In summary, the following legal and regulatory interventions should be considered in advancing the policy goal of ensuring availability of quality (generic and innovative) antimicrobials:

- Laws and regulations on standards and practices that ensure quality level is achieved (e.g. good manufacturing standards and practices);
- Legally sanctioned practices for monitoring product quality and prequalifying supplies and products (e.g. through licensing, accreditation, audit and inspection);
- Law and regulations that promote fair competition or that enable regulatory action to be taken against anti-competitive practices;
- Legally entrenching disease surveillance and management programmes; and
- Set out legal and regulatory baseline and principles for risk sharing agreements and patient access programmes.

Improving Prescribing and Dispensing

In many LMICs, antimicrobials are sold over-the-counter without a prescription or otherwise dispensed by individuals who lack professional training or authority. Even where there may be laws or regulations that proscribe such practices, they may be poorly or inadequately enforced (Singh 2017; World Health Organization 2015b). For instance, accreditation and professional licensing may not specifically target adherence to standard treatment guidelines. Consequently, the failure to adhere to guidance on responsible antimicrobial prescription would not render the healthcare provider professionally accountable or otherwise legally empower a professional body to take remedial action. Responsible prescribing and dispensing practices could also be hampered by weak healthcare infrastructure, expectations of patients and perverse financial incentives. Access to rapid or reliable diagnostic tests may be limited in a low resource health system. This could in turn encourage healthcare providers to veer towards prescribing an antibiotic in order to ensure that the prospect of a bacterial infection is addressed even if there is no reliable diagnosis to that effect. Such a conservative approach could even be a cost effective response (in the short term) if the cost of the antibiotic is lower than to order a laboratory test to validate a diagnosis (World Health Organization 2015b). For this and other reasons, providers may feel obligated to prescribe – while patients may feel entitled to use – antimicrobials, as a quick treatment option. Patients may not be aware of what appropriate use of antimicrobials means, particularly where duration of medical consultation is limited, and could consider themselves to have received substandard care if they have not been prescribed an antibiotic. At a systemic level, financial incentives may encourage overprescribing of antimicrobials. Where pharmaceutical sales generate revenue for healthcare providers and institutions, there would be a perverse financial incentive to overprescribe. Such a practice may be exacerbated where pharmaceutical companies themselves enter into profit-sharing arrangements with these providers or institutions. Additionally, it is currently impossible to determine the extent that antimicrobials are appropriately prescribed and consumed as there is a lack of reliable data across all health systems.

Laws and regulations are necessary to prohibit over-the-counter sale of antimicrobials while ensuring that patients continue to have access through appropriately trained and qualified healthcare professionals. In addition, requiring an appropriate amount of information to be indicated on packaging and to be shared as part of responsible prescribing practice could be given regulatory force. On the former, such a requirement could be taken up as a regulatory measure to ensure high-value or quality use of antimicrobials, particularly where full treatment courses are to be dispensed. Healthcare providers, institutions and professional associations have a crucial role to play in robust guideline development and implementation processes, filling evidence gaps with research, developing high-value practices, and leading or participating in efforts to shift from low-value to high-value practices. In many health systems, these stakeholders do not have sufficient or appropriate legal standing to contribute constructively to policy measure that are directed at improving prescribing and dispensing practices (Singh 2017; World Health Organization 2015b). As noted earlier, professional associations that have an interest in ensuring that standard treatment guidelines are observed by their members may not have any regulatory authority to monitor and improve such practices. Where professional organisations have the capability and motivation to improve professional practices, appropriate laws and regulations could be facilitative of this in a manner that is transparent and accountable. The challenge of perverse financial incentives is perhaps more difficult to surmount, particularly if the health system concerned is committed to particular structural arrangements or values. Legal or regulatory intervention could then be a platform for evaluation, discussion and change. For instance, legal and regulatory changes introduced by South Korea in 2000 to prohibit doctors from dispensing drugs have reduced inappropriate antibiotic prescribing (Kwon 2003; Park et al. 2005).

In summary, the following legal and regulatory interventions could be considered to improve prescribing and dispensing of antimicrobials:

- Prohibit over-the-counter sale of antimicrobials;
- Lend regulatory weight to standard treatment guidelines;

- Empower healthcare institutions and professional associations to improve prescribing and (where applicable) dispensing practices through means that include assessing provider performance;
- Introduce regulation to ensure that care is managed comprehensively;
- Laws and regulations that support implementing and monitoring policies to encourage clinically appropriate and cost-effective use of antimicrobials; and
- Evaluate, remove or manage perverse financial incentives through appropriate laws and regulations.

Ensuring Appropriate, Affordable and Equitable Access

The policy goals of ensuring appropriate, affordable and equitable access to pharmaceuticals (including antimicrobials) are aligned with the WHO's global health initiative on universal health coverage (UHC), broadly directed at promoting access for all to appropriate health services at affordable cost (World Health Assembly Resolution 2005; World Health Organization 2010a, b). Much discussion on UHC has focused on expanding populations covered by national payment systems, although comparatively little information exists on what pharmaceutical are provided, whether they meet the healthcare needs of the population, and how health systems manage pharmaceuticals so that patients receive high-value services at costs that households and systems can afford. When the types of pharmaceuticals provided do not meet population needs, risk protection is inadequate and this does not prevent household impoverishment (Yip and Hsiao 2009; Parry 2012; Wagner et al. 2008).

The economic burden of pharmaceuticals on households is high: they account for nearly half of household healthcare expenditures in 12 Asia-Pacific countries (Wagner and Ross-Degnan 2009) and for all healthcare expenses in four out of 10 households in 22 low- and 17 middle-income countries (Wagner et al. 2011). Pharmaceuticals also constitute a major source of inefficiencies in health systems. Of the ten leading sources of inefficiency in health systems identified in the 2010 World Health Report, pharmaceuticals account for the top three (World Health Organization 2010a). Underuse of generic products, use of substandard and counterfeit medicines, and inappropriate use of medicines waste scarce resources in systems. The World Health Organization estimates that more than half of all medicines globally are prescribed, dispensed, or sold inappropriately (World Health Organization 2009). For instance, overuse of antibiotics to treat acute respiratory tract infections wastes resources and leads to use of higher cost second and third line antibiotics for drug resistant infections. In many LMICs, access to a qualified healthcare professional may cost patients more time and money when compared with inappropriately or illegally obtaining antibiotics over-the-counter or from an unauthorised vendor. To promote appropriate and affordable access, national antibiotics policies and standard treatment guidelines must be supported by essential medicines lists or formularies that encourage rational and responsible use of antimicrobials. In addition, appropriate laws and regulations must be in place to ensure that the antimicrobial supply chain is secure in terms of their procurement, storage and sale (World Health Organization 2015b). These requirements extend to importation requirements and quality inspections for health systems that do not manufacture antimicrobials.

The use of antimicrobials in animals for food production or other purposes will also need to be carefully monitored and regulated. Whereas laws and regulations have conventionally been domain specific particularly in keeping regulations relating to humans distinct from nonhuman animals, the *One Health* approach endorsed in the GAP-AMR highlights the need for a more comprehensive and coordinated approach across the food, veterinary and health sectors. Many countries have yet to establish a regulatory mechanism to enforce requirements for appropriate use of antimicrobials in animals. In addition, there is inadequate infrastructure for monitoring and controlling the development of resistant pathogens in animals, their vertical transmission from one animal species to another, as well as zoonotic transmissions to humans.

Above all, WHO policy documents and guidance (2010a, 2014, 2016, 2017a) have consistently emphasised the importance of promoting equity through greater stakeholder engagement and prioritising the worst off (or otherwise the most vulnerable) in a given society. This could be especially important for decentralised health systems, where inequalities across regions may be great (see also Reid, Chap. 16, this volume). A related concern is that public awareness of appropriate antimicrobial use remains low in most, if not all, health systems. Even within healthcare institutions, infrastructure and human resources may not be adequately equipped to implement and manage infection prevention and control programmes. Equitable access as devised through paradigms such as "accountability for reasonableness" (Daniels and Sabin 2002) is arguably more likely to enable and encourage relevant stakeholders – particularly the broader community – to be interested and proactively involved in national antibiotics policies and related infection prevention and control programmes. As we shall elaborate on below, an equitable regulatory lever is crucial in support bottom-up approaches to promoting high-value use of antimicrobials (Tang et al. 2016).

In summary, the following legal and regulatory interventions could be considered to ensure appropriate, affordable and equitable access to antimicrobials:

- Introducing laws and regulations that implement and sustain infection prevention and control programmes, including appropriate surveillance mechanisms, to understand utilisation profiles, assess care seeking behaviour and barriers to care, and improve access for vulnerable populations;
- Regulation could be the basis of public awareness campaigns and continuing education for stakeholders;
- Laws and regulations may be needed to support monitoring routine medicines expenditures by therapeutic area, evaluating health technologies and budget impact, and assessing household medicines expenditure;
- Implementing and monitoring policies and programmes to reduce waste and inappropriate use through appropriate regulations;

- Requiring appropriate stakeholders' involvement or contribution through regulation; and
- Reduce the use of antibiotics as growth promoters in animals through laws and regulations.

Regulatory Lever Within a Whole-of-System Approach

In our discussion above, we have considered the different types of legal and regulatory actions or tools that could constitute the regulatory lever, taking into account pharmaceutical policy goals and the GAP-AMR regulatory principles. We have also noted that the regulatory lever is but one of other levers that are available to policy-makers, two of such levers being financial and information. In this section, we broadly explain why the regulatory lever underscores the effectiveness of these two other levers within a "whole-of-system" approach that is directed at AMR containment. By this approach, we adopt the WHO's emphasis that focus should not be limited to a particular component of a health system – broadly defined to mean "all organizations, people and actions whose primary intent is to promote, restore and maintain health"- but to recognise that different systemic components are interrelated and interact in ways that may be anticipated or unanticipated (World Health Organization 2010a; b, at p. 19).

Financial Lever

The financial lever could be thought of as being constituted by financial schemes that include budget controls, tax and incentive arrangements, and also the policies and actions of healthcare purchasers or payers, particularly social insurers (Bigdeli et al. 2014). Ideally, financing schemes should be designed to support decision-making through provision of information on demographic characteristics, health-care needs and utilisation patterns of its users, and also of healthcare providers – particularly prescribing patterns and related costs. Implementers of financial schemes exert a degree of financial control over patients and healthcare providers in terms of what they pay for, and could shape patient demand through both financial and educational means. Additionally, financial incentives should encourage cost-effective prevention and care, while financial commitments should be directed at meeting infrastructural requirement, such as surveillance mechanisms that allow the use of international and local data on disease burden and utilisation patterns to signal potential inappropriate use patterns. In reality, financial interventions, like expenditure-focused policy instruments, tend to lack specificity and often have unintended effects. For instance, a cap on funding does not necessarily encourage clinically appropriate use or otherwise reduce wasteful spending as a result of over-treatment.

Within a whole-of-system approach, the financial lever should be applied together with the regulatory lever to support the establishment of a sound information environment, by making available evidence-based clinical guidelines and economic assessments that include health technology assessment and budget impact. As we have noted above, this is crucial in overcoming the current challenge that too little information on monitoring and evaluation activities is available, primarily due to lack of mechanisms in many health systems to monitor antimicrobial prescription and use. While some information is available on how medicines are financed in these health systems, there is little information to reliably determine equitable access and appropriate use.

Information Lever

The information lever of many health systems is disproportionately focused on price rather than on appropriate use and good stewardship. There is a need to review, revise and develop information systems to collect information that will enable policy-makers to target policies that improve prescribing practices, carry out audits and conduct education programmes. Such a system should also be able combine information from different parts of the healthcare system. Regular samples of paper-based facility prescribing and dispensing records can provide information on utilization to inform policy decisions (World Health Organization 2015b).

Policies that ensure appropriate use of antibiotics in a manner that is effective, safe, equitable and efficient depend on the availability of information including population demographics, disease epidemiology, treatment approaches, and political and economic environments. Health systems will need to be capable of generating routine, up-to-date information about the type of antibiotics that are needed by patients, which antibiotics are being used and how they are used across different patient populations within the health system, who prescribed them, whether they are clinically appropriate (such as in addressing the disease burden faced by the population) and the cost spent. Without such information, it will be difficult to determine if quality of care is provided. Ideally, information systems should capture details on the antibiotics use and expenditure, along with quality of care (such as the percentage of primary care patients receiving antibiotics), and details of misuse. However, these details are usually not captured by data collection systems. For instance, where providers are paid through bundled-payment arrangements (whether case or episode-based), the information system may not be designed to capture data on the type and amount of antibiotics prescribed, since payment does not depend on such information. As we have noted above, appropriate laws and regulations could help bring about changes to information systems that prioritises AMR containment.

Constant monitoring, feedback and evaluation are important to ensure that levers continue to achieve desired goals. Crucially, member states will need to ensure that the whole-of-system approach to AMR containment could be implemented bottom-up and top-down (Elshaug et al. 2017). Bottom-up actions require stakeholders who are not in any formal positions of authority to change practices that are within their sphere of influence. Such stakeholders could be patients, clinicians, cooperatives and agricultural producers (see Schwenkenbecher, Chap. 23, this volume and Oakley, Chap.8 in this volume). In contrast, top-down actions have wider impact and the drivers of change typically include governments, professional bodies and third party payers. The use of the regulatory lever, along with other levers, should enable as well as facilitate a combination of both bottom-up and top-down actions to improve policies and practices relating to antibiotics access, use and stewardship.

Conclusion

In this chapter, we have considered how AMR containment has become a collective action problem, perhaps most comprehensively mapped out in the GAP-AMR. While the GAP-AMR itself lacks legal or regulatory force, there are at least three regulatory principles that could be drawn from it. These regulatory principles in turn require countries to adopt a variety of legal and regulatory actions or interventions that may be necessary to strengthen their regulatory lever for AMR containment. We have attempted to explicate these legal and regulatory actions in terms of four pharmaceutical policy objectives that have been articulated in a number of WHO documents and initiatives. Finally, we highlighted the crucial role of the regulatory lever in implementing the GAP-AMR, and also in enabling other levers under a whole-of-system approach.

Policies on AMR in health systems need to be responsive to shifting contexts and goals. Such adaptations must be informed by the best available evidence of what works, for whom, how and why in a given situation. In addition, routine monitoring and periodic evaluations of the impacts are necessary, and they are further crucial to ensuring quality, appropriate use and good stewardship of antimicrobials. The regulatory lever could and arguably should be applied to introduce, guide, scale-up, adapt, adjust or terminate policies on AMR containment. While it is not disputed that the regulatory lever is generally recognised to be important, there has been relatively little attention as to what it means in terms of laws and regulations that could be directed at AMR containment. If the GAP-AMR is to be effectively enabled, this lacuna that we have highlighted will require greater attention.

References

Årdal, Christine, Kevin Outterson, Steven J. Hoffman, Abdul Ghafur, Mike Sharland, Nisha Ranganathan, Richard Smith, et al. 2016. International cooperation to improve access to and sustain effectiveness of antimicrobials. *The Lancet* 387 (10015): 296–307. https://doi.org/10.1016/S0140-6736(15)00470-5.

Behdinan, Asha, Steven J. Hoffman, and Mark Pearcey. 2015. Some global policies for antibiotic resistance depend on legally binding and enforceable commitments. *The Journal of Law, Medicine & Ethics* 43 (suppl. 3): 68–73. https://doi.org/10.1111/jlme.12277.

Bigdeli, Maryam, David H. Peters, and Anita K. Wagner, eds. 2014. *Medicines in health systems: Advancing access, affordability and appropriate use*. Geneva: World Health Organization. Available at: http://www.who.int/alliance-hpsr/resources/FR_webfinal_v1.pdf.

Cheah, Phaik-Yeong, Nicholas Day, and Michael Parker. 2020. Ethics and antimalarial drug resistance. In *Ethics and drug resistance: Collective responsibility for global public health*. Cham: Springer.

Daniels, Noman, and James E. Sabin. 2002. *Setting limits fairly: Can we learn to share medical resources?* New York/Oxford: Oxford University Press.

Elshaug, Adam G., Meredith B. Rosenthal, John N. Lavis, Shannon Brownlee, Harald Schmidt, Somil Nagpal, Peter Littlejohns, Divya Srivastava, Sean Tunis, and Vikas Saini. 2017. Levers for addressing medical underuse and overuse: Achieving high-value health care. *Lancet* 390: 191–202. https://doi.org/10.1016/S0140-6736(16)32586-7.

Fleming, Alexander. 1945. Penicillin: Nobel Lecture, December 11, pp. 83–93. Available at: https://www.nobelprize.org/uploads/2018/06/fleming-lecture.pdf

Food and Agriculture Organization of the United Nations, World Organisation for Animal Health, World Health Organization. 2017. *Global framework for development & stewardship to combat antimicrobial resistance*. WHO/EMP/IAU/2017.08. Available at: http://www.who.int/phi/implementation/research/WHA_BackgroundPaper-AGlobalFrameworkDevelopmentStewardship-Version2.pdf.

G20 Leaders' Declaration: Shaping an interconnected world. Hamburg, 7/8 July. Available at: https://www.g20.org/gipfeldokumente/G20-leaders-declaration.pdf.

Haire, Bridget. 2020. Antiretrovial resistance – Ethical issues. In *Ethics and drug resistance: Collective responsibility for global public health*. Cham: Springer.

Hoffman, Steven J., and Asha Behdinan. 2016. Towards an international treaty on antimicrobial resistance. *Ottawa Law Review* 47 (2): 503. Available at: https://commonlaw.uottawa.ca/ottawa-law-review/sites/commonlaw.uottawa.ca.ottawa-law-review/files/olr_47-2_09_hoffman_behdinan_final.pdf.

Jamrozik, Euzebiusz, and Michael Selgelid. 2020. Drug-resistant infection: Causes, consequences, and responses. In *Ethics and drug resistance: Collective responsibility for global public health*. Cham: Springer.

Kwon, Soonman. 2003. Pharmaceutical reform and physician strikes in Korea: Separation of drug prescribing and dispensing. *Social Science & Medicine* 57: 529–538. https://doi.org/10.1016/S0277-9536(02)00378-7.

Leatherby, Lauren. 2017. The rise of antibiotic-resistant infections threatens economies. *Financial Times* July 7. Available at: https://www.ft.com/content/1a3b06fa-57ff-11e7-80b6-9bfa4c1f83d2.

Michael E. Porter. 2010. What Is Value in Health Care?. *New England Journal of Medicine* 363 (26): 2477–2481

Park, Sylvia, Stephen B. Soumerai, Alyce S. Adams, Jonathan A. Finkelstein, Sunmee Jang, and Dennis Ross-Degnan. 2005. Antibiotic use following a Korean national policy to prohibit medication dispensing by physicians. *Health Policy and Planning* 20 (5): 302–309. https://doi.org/10.1093/heapol/czi033.

Parry, Jane. 2012. Nine of 10 Chinese are covered by medical insurance, but access to treatment remains a problem. *BMJ* 344: e248. https://doi.org/10.1136/bmj.e248.

Public Health England. 2015. *Health matters: Antimicrobial resistance*. Available at: https://www.gov.uk/government/publications/health-matters-antimicrobial-resistance/health-matters-antimicrobial-resistance.

Reid, Lynette. 2020. Antimicrobial resistance and social inequalities in health: Considerations of justice. In *Ethics and drug resistance: Collective responsibility for global public health*. Cham: Springer.

Reinl, James. 2016. UN declaration on antimicrobial resistance lacks targets. *The Lancet* 388 (10052): 1365. https://doi.org/10.1016/S0140-6736(16)31769-X.

Review on Antimicrobial Resistance. 2014. *Antimicrobial resistance: Tackling a crisis for the health and wealth of nations*. Available at: http://www.jpiamr.eu/wp-content/uploads/2014/12/AMR-Review-Paper-Tackling-a-crisis-for-the-health-and-wealth-of-nations_1-2.pdf.

Rogers Van Katwyk, Susan, Marie Evelyne Danik, Ioana Pantis, Rachel Smith, John-Arne Røttingen, and Steven J. Hoffman. 2016. Developing an approach to assessing the political feasibility of global collective action and an international agreement on antimicrobial resistance. *Global Health Research and Policy* 1 (1): 20. https://doi.org/10.1186/s41256-016-0020-9.

Scheuber, Andrew. 2017. *Angela Merkel discusses global antibiotic challenge with Imperial academic*. Imperial College London. Available at: http://www3.imperial.ac.uk/newsandeventspggrp/imperialcollege/newssummary/news_23-2-2017-15-42-19.

Singh, Poonam. 2017. One health approach to tackle antimicrobial resistance in South East Asia. *BMJ* 358: 3625. https://doi.org/10.1136/bmj.j3625.

Smith, Richard D., and Joanna Coast. 2002. Antimicrobial resistance: A global response. *Bulletin of the World Health Organization* 80 (2): 126–133. Available at: http://www.who.int/iris/handle/10665/71062.

Tang, Yuqing, Chaojie Liu, and Xinping Zhang. 2016. Public reporting as a prescriptions quality improvement measure in primary care settings in China: Variations in effects associated with diagnoses. *Scientific Reports* 6: 39361. https://doi.org/10.1038/srep39361.

United Nations. 2015. *Transforming our world: The 2030 agenda for sustainable development*. A/RES/70/1. Available at: https://sustainabledevelopment.un.org/content/documents/21252030%20Agenda%20for%20Sustainable%20Development%20web.pdf.

———. 2016. *Press release: High-level meeting on antimicrobial resistance*. Available at: http://www.un.org/pga/71/2016/09/21/press-release-hl-meeting-on-antimicrobial-resistance/.

United Nations News Centre. 2016. *At UN, global leaders commit to act on antimicrobial resistance*. September 21. Available at: http://www.un.org/apps/news/story.asp?NewsID=55011#.WcDFn9FpHb0.

Wagner, Anita K., and Dennis Ross-Degnan. 2009. The potential for insurance systems to increase access to and appropriate use of medicines in Asia-Pacific countries. In *Prescribing cultures and pharmaceutical policy in the Asia-Pacific*, ed. Karen Eggleston. Stanford: Walter H. Shorenstein Asia-Pacific Research Center.

Wagner, Anita K., Madeleine Valera, Amy J. Graves, Sheila Laviña, and Dennis Ross-Degnan. 2008. Costs of hospital care for hypertension in an insured population without an outpatient medicines benefit: An observational study in the Philippines. *BMC Health Services Research* 8: 161. https://doi.org/10.1186/1472-6963-8-161.

Wagner, Anita K., Amy J. Graves, Sheila K. Reiss, Robert LeCates, Fang Zhang, and Dennis Ross-Degnan. 2011. Access to care and medicines, burden of health care expenditures, and risk protection: Results from the World Health Survey. *Health Policy* 100 (2–3): 151–158. https://doi.org/10.1016/j.healthpol.2010.08.004.

Wernli, Didier, Thomas Haustein, John Conly, Yehuda Carmeli, Ilona Kickbusch, and Stephan Harbarth. 2011. A call for action: The application of the international health regulations to the global threat of antimicrobial resistance. *PLoS Medicine* 8 (4): e1001022. https://doi.org/10.1371/journal.pmed.1001022.

World Bank. 2017. *Drug-resistant infections: A threat to our economic future*. Washington, DC: World Bank. Available at: http://documents.worldbank.org/curated/en/455311493396671601/pdf/114679-REVISED-v1-Drug-Resistant-Infections-Executive-Summary.pdf.

World Health Assembly Resolution. 2005. *WHA58.33 – Sustainable health financing, universal coverage and social health insurance*. WHA Resolution: Fifty-eighth World Health Assembly. Available at: http://apps.who.int/medicinedocs/documents/s21475en/s21475en.pdf.

———. 2015a. *Antimicrobial resistance: Draft global action plan on antimicrobial resistance*. A68/20. Available at: http://apps.who.int/gb/ebwha/pdf_files/WHA68/A68_20-en.pdf.

———. 2015b. *WHA68.7 – Global action plan on antimicrobial resistance*. WHA Resolution: Sixty-eighth World Health Assembly. Available at: http://apps.who.int/medicinedocs/en/d/Js21889en/.

World Health Organization. 1985. *The rational use of drugs: Report of the conference of experts. Nairobi, 25-28 November 1985*. Geneva: World Health Organization. Available at: http://apps.who.int/medicinedocs/documents/s17054e/s17054e.pdf.

———. 2001. *WHO global strategy for containment of antimicrobial resistance*. Geneva: World Health Organization. Available at: http://www.who.int/drugresistance/WHO_Global_Strategy_English.pdf.

———. 2009. *Medicines use in primary care in developing and transitional countries*. Geneva: World Health Organization. Available at: http://www.who.int/medicines/publications/who_emp_2009.3/en/index.html.

———. 2010a. *The world health report. Health systems financing: The path to universal coverage*. Geneva: World Health Organization. Available at: http://www.who.int/whr/2010/en/index.html.

———. 2010b. *Western Pacific Regional strategy for health systems based on the values of primary health care*. Available at: http://www.wpro.who.int/topics/health_systems/wpro_strategy_health_systems_primary_health_care.pdf.

———. 2012a. *Governance for health in the 21st century*. Geneva: World Health Organization. Available at: http://www.euro.who.int/__data/assets/pdf_file/0019/171334/RC62BD01-Governance-for-Health-Web.pdf.

———. 2012b. *The pursuit of responsible use of medicines: Sharing and learning from country experiences*. Geneva: World Health Organization. Available at: http://apps.who.int/iris/bitstream/10665/75828/1/WHO_EMP_MAR_2012.3_eng.pdf.

———. 2014. *Making fair choices on the path to universal health coverage*. Geneva: World Health Organization. Available at: http://www.who.int/choice/documents/making_fair_choices/en/.

———. 2015a. *Global action plan on antimicrobial resistance*. Geneva: World Health Organization. Available at: http://www.who.int.libproxy1.nus.edu.sg/antimicrobial-resistance/publications/global-action-plan/en/.

———. 2015b. *Antimicrobial resistance in the Western Pacific Region: A review of surveillance and health systems response*. Geneva: World Health Organization. Available at: http://www.wpro.who.int/entity/drug_resistance/documents/amr_wpr.pdf.

———. 2016. *Health care without avoidable infections: The critical role of infection prevention and control*. Geneva: World Health Organization. Available at: http://apps.who.int.libproxy1.nus.edu.sg/iris/bitstream/10665/246235/1/WHO-HIS-SDS-2016.10-eng.pdf.

———. 2017a. *Health emergencies represent some of the greatest risks to the global economy and security: Remarks delivered by Dr Tedros Adhanom Ghebreyesus to G20 8 July 2017*. Available at: http://www.who.int/dg/speeches/2017/g20-summit/en/.

———. 2017b. *Report of the 21st WHO expert committee on the selection and use of essential medicines*. Geneva: World Health Organization. Available at: http://www.who.int/medicines/publications/essentialmedicines/EML_2017_ExecutiveSummary.pdf?ua=1.

———. 2017c. *WHO global surveillance and monitoring system for substandard and falsified medical products*. Geneva: World Health Organization. Available at: https://www.who.int/medicines/regulation/ssffc/publications/gsms-report-sf/en/.

———. n.d. *About WHO: What we do*. Available at: http://www.who.int/about/what-we-do/en/.

Yip, Winnie, and William C. Hsiao. 2009. Non-evidence-based policy: How effective is China's new cooperative medical scheme in reducing medical impoverishment? *Social Science and Medicine* 68: 201–209. https://doi.org/10.1016/j.socscimed.2008.09.066.

12

The Super-Wicked Problem of Antimicrobial Resistance

Jasper Littmann, A. M. Viens, and Diego S. Silva

Keywords Complex systems · Social policy · Bioethics · Political philosophy

Antimicrobial resistance (AMR) – the progressive process by which microbes, such as bacteria, through evolutionary, environmental and social factors develop the ability to become resistant to drugs that were once effective at treating them – is a threat from which no one can escape. It is one of the largest threats to clinical and global health in the twenty-first century – inflicting monumental health, economic and social consequences.[1] All persons locally and globally, and even all future persons yet to come into existence, all suffer the shared, interdependent vulnerability to this threat that will have a substantial impact on all aspects of our lives. For example,

[1] J O'Neill, et al., *Infection Prevention, Control and Surveillance: Limiting the Development and Spread of Drug Resistance* (London: Review on Antimicrobial Resistance, 2016) https://amr-review.org/sites/default/files/Health%20infrastructure%20and%20surveillance%20final%20version_LR_NO%20CROPS.pdf (accessed September 29, 2017); President's Council of Advisors on Science and Technology, *Report To The President On Combating Antimicrobial Resistance* (Washington: PCAST, 2014); World Health Organization, *The Evolving Threat of Antimicrobial Resistance: Options for Action* (Geneva: WHO Press, 2012); World Economic Forum, *Global Risks 2013 – Insight Report, Eighth Edition* (Geneva, 2013); S.C. Davies, J. Grant and M. Catchpole, *The Drugs Don't Work: A Global Threat* (London: Penguin, 2013); O.O. Adeyi, et al., *Drug-Resistant Infections: A Threat to Our Economic Future* (Washington, DC: World Bank, 2017).

J. Littmann (✉)
Norwegian Institute of Public Health, Oslo, Norway
e-mail: jasper.littmann@fhi.no

A. M. Viens
School of Global Health, York University, Toronto, Canada
e-mail: amviens@yorku.ca

D. S. Silva
Sydney Health Ethics, School of Public Health, University of Sydney, Sydney, NSW, Australia
e-mail: diego.silva@sydney.edu.au

while reliable data are hard to find, the European Centre for Disease Prevention and Control (ECDC) has conservatively estimated that, in Europe alone, AMR causes additional annual cost to health care systems of at least €1.5 billion, and is responsible for around 25,000 deaths per year. Furthermore, AMR significantly increases the cost of treating bacterial infections with an increase in length of hospital stays and average number of re-consultations, as well as the resultant lost productivity from increased morbidity.[2] With a combined cost of up to $100 trillion to the global economy – pushing a further 28 million people into extreme poverty – this is one of the most pressing challenges facing the world.[3] Most troublingly, if we do not succeed in diminishing the progression of AMR, there is the very real potential for it to threaten common procedures and treatments of modern medicine, including the safety and efficacy of surgical procedures and immunosuppressing chemotherapy.[4] Some experts are warning that we may soon be ushering in a post-antibiotic area.[5]

Challenges in Responding to AMR

There exists a multitude of policy responses to AMR at the local, national and international levels.[6] Unfortunately, their success to date has only been limited.[7] This may partly be due to the fact that many microorganisms are highly adaptable and constantly evolving, thereby presenting a perpetual challenge to clinicians, researchers, public health professionals and policy-makers.[8] However, the formulation and

---

[2] L.L. Maragakis, E.N. Perencevich and S.E. Cosgrove, 'Clinical and Economic Burden of Antimicrobial Resistance,' *Expert Review of Anti-infective Therapy* 6(2008): 751–63; F. Alam, et al. 'The additional costs of antibiotics and re-consultations for antibiotic-resistant Escherichia coli urinary tract infections managed in general practice,' *International Journal of Antimicrobial Agents* 33(2009): 255–57; R. Smith and J. Coast, 'The true cost of antimicrobial resistance,' *BMJ* 2013; 346: f1493; Centers of Disease Control and Prevention, *Antibiotic Resistance Threats in the United States, 2013* (Atlanta: Centers of Disease Control and Prevention, 2013)

[3] J. O'Neill et al., *Tackling Drug-Resistant Infections Globally: Final Report and Recommendations* (London: Review on Antimicrobial Resistance, 2016), available at https://amr-review.org/sites/default/files/160518_Final%20paper_with%20cover.pdf (accessed September 29, 2017).

[4] A. Teillant, S. Gandra, D. Barter, D.J. Morgan, and R. Laxminarayan, 'Potential burden of antibiotic resistance on surgery and cancer chemotherapy antibiotic prophylaxis in the USA: a literature review and modelling study,' *Lancet Infectious Diseases* 15(2015): 1429–37.

[5] S.C. Davies, J. Grant and M. Catchpole, *The Drugs Don't Work: A Global Threat* (London: Penguin, 2013).

[6] World Health Organization, *Global Strategy for Containment of Antimicrobial Resistance* (Geneva: WHO, 2001); Infectious Diseases Society of America, 'The 10 × '20 Initiative: Pursuing a Global Commitment to Develop 10 New Antibacterial Drugs by 2020,' *Clinical Infectious Diseases* 8(2010): 1081–83; Bundesministerium für Gesundheit, *Deutsche Antibiotikaresistenz-Strategie* (Berlin, 2011); Department of Health, *UK Five Year Antimicrobial Resistance Strategy 2013 to 2018* (London, 2013)

[7] World Health Organization, *Antimicrobial Resistance – Global Report on Surveillance* (Geneva: WHO Press, 2014)

[8] A.S. Fauci and D.M. Morens, 'The Perpetual Challenge of Infectious Diseases,' *New England Journal of Medicine* 366(2012): 454–61.

implementation of effective polices are also compounded by the complexity of the challenge. This complexity pertains to the number of local, national and international stakeholders involved, the difficulty in establishing successful collaboration and coordination mechanisms across different policy areas, and the numerous interrelated drivers that make this a problem at the global scale.[9]

The number of stakeholders who contribute to the emergence of AMR is extraordinarily large.[10] Misuse and over-prescription of antibiotics, for example, are driven not only by health care professionals but also consumers – many of whom will not use antibiotics as instructed, often without being aware of the potential consequences of their actions.[11] Other patient groups entirely lack access to appropriate antimicrobial treatment, especially in poorer or less developed settings.[12] Where treatment is either unaffordable for many or infrastructure is lacking, people are more likely to self-medicate or buy counterfeit drugs through unofficial channels, increasing the chance that their drugs are less effective or unsuitable for treating the infection.[13] Beyond human usage, the pervasive use of antibiotics outside of medical settings also remains a key source of resistance. Indeed, it is estimated that more antibiotics are given to animals than consumed by humans – and, in many instances, for non-therapeutic use.[14] The wide use of antibiotics within agricultural, aquaculture, horticultural and animal farming industries all provide multiple opportunities for the increase incidence and prevalence of antibiotic-resistant bacteria.[15]

AMR does not, therefore, squarely fall into a single policy domain and any effective policy will require collaboration among a wide range of experts, such as clinicians, veterinarians, microbiologists, pharmacologists, epidemiologists, lawyers,

---

[9] R. Laximinarayan, et al., 'Antibiotic resistance - the need for global solutions,' *Lancet Infectious Diseases* 13(2013): 1057–98.

[10] W. Albrich, D. Monnet, S. Harbarth, 'Antibiotic Selection Pressure and Resistance in Streptococcus pneumoniae and Streptococcus pyogenes,' *Emerging Infectious Diseases* 10(2004): 514–17.

[11] C.C. Butler, et al., 'Understanding the culture of prescribing: qualitative study of general practitioners' and patients' perceptions of antibiotics for sore throat,' *BMJ* 317(1998): 637–42; I. Björkman, et al., 'Infectious disease management in primary care: perceptions of GPs.' BMC Fam Pract, 12:1 (2011); N. Britten, 'Patients' expectations of consultations', *BMJ*, 328 (2004):416–17

[12] M. Mendelson, et al. 'Maximising access to achieve appropriate human antimicrobial use in low-income and middle-income countries,' *Lancet* 387(2015):188–98; R. Laxminarayan, et al., 'Access to effective antimicrobials: a worldwide challenge,' *Lancet* 387(2016): 168–175.

[13] N. Gualde, *Resistance: The human struggle against infection* (New York: Dana Press, 2006); R. Laxminarayan and D.L. Heymann, 'Challenges of drug resistance in the developing world,' *BMJ* 344(2012): e1567.

[14] J. O'Neill, et al., *Antimicrobials in agriculture and the environment: reducing unnecessary use and waste* (London: Review on Antimicrobial Resistance, 2016) https://amr-review.org/sites/default/files/Antimicrobials%20in%20agriculture%20and%20the%20environment%20-%20Reducing%20unnecessary%20use%20and%20waste.pdf (accessed September 12, 2017).

[15] Food and Agriculture Organization of the United Nations, *Drivers, Dynamics and Epidemiology of Antimicrobial Resistance in Animal Production* (Geneva: WHO, 2016); R.W. Meek RW, H. Vyas and L.J.V. Piddock, 'Nonmedical Uses of Antibiotics: Time to Restrict Their Use?' *PLoS Biology* 13(2015): e1002266. https://doi.org/10.1371/journal.pbio.1002266.

philosophers, economists and public health professionals.[16] This requires high degrees of multi-sectorial integration, coordination and accountability mechanisms, for which existing policy-making structures are inappropriate or insufficient.[17] This is further compounded by the fact that AMR has numerous interdependent biological and social drivers that make it a problem on the global scale. Expanding international travel, tourism and trade will continue to perpetuate resistance beyond current levels.[18] As such, while national and regional policies can certainly impact on the prevalence of drug-resistant infections,[19] the global dissemination of resistant bacteria demonstrate why such localised efforts alone cannot be ultimately effective.[20]

As a result of all of these considerations, AMR also raises distinctive ethical issues, which must not only be accounted for in our policy and response activities, but will play an important role in supporting the numerous difficult choices involved in balancing the benefits and burdens associated with protecting antibiotic effectiveness and reducing the spread of drug-resistant infections.[21] Our traditional normative theories and principles, as developed in other infection prevention and control contexts, will be insufficient if mechanically applied as if it were just another problem of infectious disease ethics. It will require careful attention to the morally-relevant features of what makes AMR a distinctive problem, and due care and context-specificity in the application of moral guidance and regulation. The ethical analysis required to shape and guide our policy response to the problem of AMR

---

[16] S.B. Levy, *The Antibiotic Paradox* (Cambridge, MA: Perseus Publishing, 2002).

[17] R.D. Smith and J. Coast, 'Antimicrobial resistance: a global response,' *Bulletin of the World Health Organization* 80(2002): 126–133; R. Laxminarayan, et al., 'Antibiotic resistance-the need for global solutions,' *Lancet Infectious Diseases* 13(2013): 1057–98; C. Årdal, et al., 'International cooperation to improve access to and sustain effectiveness of antimicrobials,' *Lancet* 387(2015): 296–307; S. J. Hoffman and T. Ottersen, 'Addressing Antibiotic Resistance Requires Robust International Accountability Mechanisms,' *The Journal of Law, Medicine and Ethics* 43(2015): 53–64.

[18] D.W. MacPherson, B.D. Gushulak and W.B. Baine, 'Population Mobility, Globalization, and Antimicrobial Drug Resistance,' *Emerging Infectious Diseases* 17(2009): 1727–1732; Z. S. Ahammad, et al., 'Increased Waterborne blaNDM-1 Resistance Gene Abundances Associated with Seasonal Human Pilgrimages to the Upper Ganges River,' *Environmental Science & Technology* 48(2014): 3014–3020; A.H. Holmes, L.S. Moore and A. Sundsfjord, 'Understanding the mechanisms and drivers of antimicrobial resistance,' *Lancet* 387(2016): 176–87.

[19] For instance, as illustrated by the significant variation in the proportion of methicillin-resistant Staphylococcus aureus (MRSA) infections across European hospitals. See, e.g., European Centre for Disease Prevention and Control, *Annual epidemiological report on communicable diseases in Europe* (Stockholm: ECDC, 2011).

[20] I.N. Okeke and R. Edelman, 'Dissemination of Antibiotic-Resistant Bacteria across Geographic Borders,' *Clinical Infectious Diseases* 33(2001): 364–369; S.E. Majowicz, et al., 'The Global Burden of Nontyphoidal *Salmonella* Gastroenteritis,' *Clin Infect Dis* 50(2010): 882–89; L.S. Tzouvelekis, et al., 'Carbapenemases in Klebsiella pneumoniae and Other Enterobacteriaceae: an Evolving Crisis of Global Dimensions,' *Clinical Microbiology Reviews*. 25(2012): 682–707; Nicola K. Petty, et al. 'Global dissemination of a multidrug resistant Escherichia coli clone,' *PNAS* 111(2014): 5694–5699.

[21] J. Littmann and A.M. Viens, 'The Ethical Significance of Antimicrobial Resistance,' *Public Health Ethics* 8(2015): 209–224.

also necessitates thinking and theorizing that is able to incorporate and reflect the various biological, social, political and legal factors involved in the spread and control of drug-resistant infections.

In this paper, we will argue that the concept of super-wicked problems can provide an apt description of the current situation regarding AMR, and that it will help us better understand some of the complex ethical challenges associated with AMR. Furthermore, framing AMR as a super-wicked problem will help to explain why at first glance, AMR appears to be so similar to other large policy challenges, such as climate change. However, we will argue that the structural similarity should not lead us to conclude that attempts to mitigate one super-wicked problem can simply be transferred to another. Instead, we suggest that the crucial feature of super-wicked problems is the need to change *path dependency* – a term we will explain more fully below – and that this change will likely require unique approaches, methods and tools for each super-wicked problem. To develop this argument, we will first introduce the ideas of super-wicked problems as a way to frame AMR. Second, we will argue that conceptualizing AMR as a super-wicked problem can help inform policy making by highlighting how our efforts should be focused. Finally, in sections four and five, we provide a potential way to move forward, and highlight key ethical issues that arise in this context.

Framing AMR as a Super-Wicked Problem

The concept of wicked problems, which has its origins in Rittel and Webber's paper about planning theory, describes certain policy problems as complex challenges that do not respond to standard problem-solving mechanisms.[22] Rittel and Webber suggest that the success of social policy in the 19th and early twentieth century was essentially the picking of low-hanging fruits, and that the policy challenges that societies are now facing are much more difficult to address.[23] Inherent complexity (i.e., the overlapping and varied sources of influence or causes to a social problem that resist simple linear solutions),[24] inter-relatedness with other policy fields, and several conflicting goals that might each be reasonably pursued, make some policy problems "wicked". According to Rittel and Webber, these problems are not solvable by traditional instruments of policy making, especially not by cost-benefit or

22 H.W.J. Rittel and M.M. Webber, 'Dilemmas in a General Theory of Planning,' *Policy Sciences* 4:2 (1973): 155–69.

23 H.W.J. Rittel and M.M. Webber, 'Dilemmas in a General Theory of Planning,' *Policy Sciences* 4:2 (1973): 155–69.

24 M.C. Jackson, *Systems Thinking: Creative Holism for Managers* (West Sussex, UK: John Wiley and Sons, Ltd., 2003).

system analysis, as these approaches cannot make sense of all dimensions of wicked problems.[25]

Wicked problems are characterized by the fact that proposed solutions cannot be judged as 'right' or 'wrong' but merely as more or less suitable, and they do not allow for a trial-and-error approach to policy-making. Instead, Rittel and Webber argue, wicked problems only allow policy-makers a single shot at solving the problem – if this fails, the unsuccessful policy will have changed the original problem to such an extent its initial alternatives may no longer be viable contenders.[26]

The concept of wicked problems has been applied to a number of areas as diverse as coastal governance,[27] liberal arts and design[28] and, more recently, climate change. It has been argued, however, that the latter no longer presents a wicked, but a 'super-wicked' problem.[29] Super-wicked problems provide an even greater challenge due to four additional complications that policy makers have to engage with. These criteria are:

(i) Time for finding a solution to a policy challenge is running out;
(ii) Those seeking to solve the problem are part of the cause;
(iii) Central authorities to address the problem are either weak or non-existent; and
(iv) Policy responses discount the future irrationally.[30]

The following section illustrates how these criteria can be applied to the case of AMR, why it should be viewed as a super-wicked problem and how each aspect of the problem raises important ethical concerns that must be factored into how we will be justified in responding to AMR as a super-wicked problem.

Criterion 1: Time Is Running Out

Super-wicked problems require drastic and urgent responses if they are not to become unsolvable policy dilemmas. In the case of AMR, it is evident that increasing drug resistance will exacerbate the existing challenge, which has led to concerns

[25] H.W.J. Rittel and M.M. Webber, 'Dilemmas in a General Theory of Planning,' *Policy Sciences* 4:2 (1973): 155–69.

[26] H.W.J. Rittel and M.M. Webber, 'Dilemmas in a General Theory of Planning,' *Policy Sciences* 4:2 (1973): 155–69.

[27] S. Jentoft and R. Chuenpagdee, 'Fisheries and coastal governance as a wicked problem,' *Marine Policy* 33(2009): 553–60.

[28] R. Buchanan, 'Wicked Problems in Design Thinking,' *Design Issues* 8(1992): 5–21.

[29] R. Lazarus, 'Super wicked problems and climate change: restraining the present to liberate the future,' *Cornell Law Review* 94(2009): 1153–234; K. Levin, et al., 'Overcoming the tragedy of super wicked problems: constraining our future selves to ameliorate global climate change,' *Policy Sciences* 45:2 (2012): 123–52.

[30] K. Levin, et al., 'Overcoming the tragedy of super wicked problems: constraining our future selves to ameliorate global climate change,' *Policy Sciences* 45:2 (2012): 123–52.

about a "post-antibiotic era".[31] There is thus, in short, an observable trend towards more complex cases of AMR, which will either be very difficult to treat or no longer respond to antibiotics at all.[32] Indeed, for some infections, such as tuberculosis or gonorrhea, resistance to all common treatments can already be observed.[33] As multi- and extensively drug resistant infections are being registered more and more frequently and with a lack of new antibiotics under development, the prospect of total antimicrobial resistance is no longer an abstract worst-case scenario.[34] This not only signals the need to make exigent decisions about a large and serious risk of harm for individuals and populations, but also factoring in the ethics of acting under conditions of necessity, urgency and uncertainty – and how this may differ from policy responses taken under conditions of normalcy.[35]

Criterion 2: Those Seeking a Solution Are Part of the Problem

AMR is a multi-factorial problem and often those involved in combating it also contribute to, or exacerbate it, in some important way:

- *Health care professionals,* who in many countries act as gatekeepers for access to antibiotics, often prescribe more antibiotics than necessary, which can lead to higher prevalence of drug-resistant infections.[36] There in an increasing number of studies, which indicate that a high proportion of prescriptions of antibiotics do not comply with scientific guidelines.[37] Furthermore, appropriate infection

---

[31] N. Brown, 'Dawn of the post-antibiotic age?' *BMJ* 309(1994): 615; A.J. Alanis, 'Resistance to Antibiotics: Are We in the Post-Antibiotic Era?' *Arch Med Res* 36(2005): 687–705.

[32] European Centre for Disease Prevention and Control, *Antimicrobial resistance surveillance in Europe: Annual report of the European Antimicrobial Resistance Surveillance Network (EARS-Net) 2011* (Stockholm, 2012).

[33] E. Alirol, et al., 'Multidrug-resistant gonorrhea: A research and development roadmap to discover new medicines,' *PLoS Med* 14(2017): e1002366; World Health Organization, *Treatment guidelines for drug-resistant tuberculosis, 2016 update* (Geneva: WHO, October 2016 revision) http://apps.who.int/iris/bitstream/10665/250125/1/9789241549639-eng.pdf?ua=1&ua=1 (Accessed September 25, 2017).

[34] European Centre for Disease Prevention and Control, *The bacterial challenge: time to react* (Stockholm, 2009).

[35] See, e.g., A.M. Viens, 'Normative Uncertainty and the Ethics of Risk Regulation in Emergency,' in A. Alemanno (ed.), *Governing Disasters: The Challenges of Emergency Risk Regulation* (Edward Elgar Publishing, 2011), pp. 137–46; A.M. Viens, *In Extremis: Morality in Times of Emergency* (London: University of London PhD, 2012).

[36] R.G. Finch, 'Antibiotic resistance: a view from the prescriber,' *Nature Reviews Microbiology* 2(2004): 989–94; V.I. Enne, 'Reducing antimicrobial resistance in the community by restricting prescribing: can it be done?' *Journal of Antimicrobial Chemotherapy* 65(2010): 179–82.

[37] K.E. Fleming-Dutra, A.L. Hersh and D.J. Shapiro, 'Prevalence of Inappropriate Antibiotic Prescriptions Among US Ambulatory Care Visits, 2010–2011,' *JAMA* 315(2016): 1864–1873. doi:https://doi.org/10.1001/jama.2016.4151.

prevention and control can reduce the need for antibiotics in the first place – which is an area where improvements can be made too.[38]

- *Pharmaceutical companies* have steadily decreased research efforts into new antimicrobial drugs, despite mounting pressures on health care systems to introduce new and effective drugs. The lack of investment is, at least, partly caused by concerns over limited returns on investment due to advancing AMR.[39] Margaret Chan, former World Health Organization (WHO) Director-General, recently alluded to this problem, when she rhetorically asked: "[f]rom an industry perspective, why invest considerable sums of money to develop a new antimicrobial when irrational use will accelerate its ineffectiveness before the R&D investment can be recouped?"[40] Recent advances in clinical research show that it may be possible to develop entirely new classes of antibiotics.[41] However, the time frame for their development remains unclear and unless novel ways of financing are introduced, their prices are likely to be prohibitive for most patients in low and middle-income countries (LMICs). The industry perspective is that the investment into new antibiotics is only financially feasible, if considerable lump sum payments, so-called market entry rewards, are paid out. These are usually estimated to have to be greater than $ 1 billion.[42] Moreover, the antibiotic production process and discarded antibiotic-laced waste can also have a considerably negative environmental impact that further perpetuates resistance.[43]

---

[38] J. O'Neill et al., *Tackling Drug-Resistant Infections Globally: Final Report and Recommendations* (London: Review on Antimicrobial Resistance, 2016), available at https://amr-review.org/sites/default/files/160518_Final%20paper_with%20cover.pdf (accessed September 29, 2017).

[39] C. Morel and E. Mossialos, 'Stoking the antibiotic pipeline,' *BMJ* 340(2010): c2115.

[40] M. Chan, *Secondary Antimicrobial Resistance in the European Union and the World* (Geneva: World Health Organization, 2012), available at: http://www.who.int/dg/speeches/2012/amr_20120314/en/ (accessed September 29, 2017).

[41] L.L. Ling, et al., 'A new antibiotic kills pathogens without detectable resistance,' *Nature* 517(2015): 455–59.

[42] R. Laxminarayan, P. Matsoso, S Pant, C. Brower, J.A. Røttingen, K. Klugman and S. Davies, 'Access to effective antimicrobials: a worldwide challenge,' *Lancet* 387(2016): 168–175; K. Outterson, et al., 'Delinking Investment in Antibiotic Research and Development from Sales Revenues: The Challenges of Transforming a Promising Idea into Reality,' *PLOS Medicine* 13(2016): e1002043. https://doi.org/10.1371/journal.pmed.1002043.

[43] K.D. Brown, et al., 'Occurrence of antibiotics in hospital, residential, and dairy effluent, municipal wastewater, and the Rio Grande in New Mexico,' *Science of the Total Environment* 366(2006): 772–783; J. Fick, et al., 'Contamination of surface, ground, and drinking water from pharmaceutical production,' *Environ Toxicol Chem* 28(2009): 2522–7; D.G.J. Larsson, 'Pollution from drug manufacturing: review and perspectives. *Phil. Trans. R. Soc. B* 369(2014): 20130571; Changing Markets Foundation, *Superbugs in the Supply Chain: How Pollution from Antibiotics Factories in India and China is Fuelling the Global Rise of Drug-Resistant Infections* (Utrecht: Changing Markets Foundation, 2016); R. Laxminarayan and R.R. Chaudhury, 'Antibiotic Resistance in India: Drivers and Opportunities for Action,' *PLoS Medicine* 3(2016): e1001974; C. Lübbert, et al., 'Environmental pollution with antimicrobial agents from bulk drug manufacturing industries in Hyderabad, South India, is associated with dissemination of extended-spectrum beta-lactamase and carbapenemase-producing pathogens,' *Infection* 45(2017): 479–491.

- *Patients* who are prescribed antibiotics often fail to adhere to treatment recommendations. This problem is exacerbated in countries where antibiotics are available for purchase over the counter, and patients may be unable to afford or have access to a health care professional who can prescribe and dispense the appropriate drug.[44]
- *Food Producers and Sellers* must continue to take significant steps to reduce the use of antibiotics as growth promoters and adopt practices that reduce the extent to which the food chain continues to be a key pathway for the transmission of resistant pathogens.[45] We also need to ensure AMR surveillance systems include resistance levels in animal stocks and food systems.
- *Governments and intergovernmental organizations* still lack the requisite regulation and governance structures to address the complexity associated with AMR and remain focused on multilateral and bilateral agreements that were commonly used in the middle of the twentieth century.[46]

The various and complex interacting contributions to the spread of AMR make it difficult (though certainly not impossible) to attribute causal responsibility to past action, including a failure to act. This also raises important questions about how our policy response should hold individuals, groups and institutions morally responsible for their complicity or causal contribution to AMR in any accountability mechanisms developed going forward.

Criterion 3: Central Authorities to Address the Problem Are either Weak or Non-existent

There is currently a lack of institutional structures that can meet the challenge of AMR effectively and at all policy levels. While international organizations, such as WHO or ECDC, have developed guidelines for prudent use of antibiotics, as well as

[44] M.B. Planta, 'The Role of Poverty in Antimicrobial Resistance' *J Am Board Fam Med*, 20:6 (2007):533–39; I.N. Okeke, A. Lamikanra, R. Edelman, 'Socioeconomic and behavioral factors leading to acquired bacterial resistance to antibiotics in developing countries,' *Emerging Infectious Diseases* 5(1999): 18–27; D.J. Morgan, I.N. Okeke, R. Laxminarayan, E.N. Perencevich and S. Weisenberg, 'Non-prescription antimicrobial use worldwide: a systematic review,' *The Lancet Infectious Diseases* 11(2011): 692–701.

[45] C. Verraes, et al., 'Antimicrobial Resistance in the Food Chain: A Review,' *International Journal of Environmental Research and Public Health* 10(2013): 2643–2669; T. P. Van Boeckel, et al., 'Global trends in antimicrobial use in food animals,' *Proceedings of the National Academy of Sciences of the United States of America* 112(2015): 5649–5654; T. P. Van Boeckel, et al. 'Reducing antimicrobial use in food animals,' *Science* 357(2017): 1350–1352.

[46] A. C. Singer, et al. 'Review of Antimicrobial Resistance in the Environment and Its Relevance to Environmental Regulators,' *Frontiers in Microbiology* 7(2016):1728; Gabriel Birgand, et al., 'Comparison of governance approaches for the control of antimicrobial resistance: Analysis of three European countries,' *Antimicrobial Resistance & Infection Control* 7(2018): 28. More is written regarding the role of these stakeholders below, under criterion 3.

programs for co-operation and data sharing, their implementation lies with the respective national governments and adherence cannot be enforced.[47] Failure to follow these recommendations is not necessarily a matter of ignorance or antipathy – in many instances countries may simply lack the control mechanisms, infrastructure, expertise, or resources to meet all requirements and recommendations of best-practice guidelines. It is also being increasingly recognized that poor governance and political corruption make major contributions to our inability to effectively respond to AMR.[48] However, since drug resistance cannot be confined by national borders, these discrepancies and deficiencies in national health systems and policies inevitably threatens the effectiveness of antibiotics and control of drug-resistant infections, even in countries that strictly enforce measures to reduce and control the use of antibiotics and mitigate the spread of AMR. More recently, the United Nations has sought to address AMR more comprehensively across sectors and policy areas, both by establishing a temporary interagency coordination group, and by strengthening the tripartite, a coordinating forum comprised of WHO, FAO, OIE, and UN Environment.[49] Nevertheless, coordination between international mechanisms and national institutions remains a voluntary process, for which few dedicated resources are available.

This raises important questions about, for instance, who should take ultimate responsibility for antimicrobial stewardship when there are no central authorities or where jurisdictions lack the resources or infrastructure to undertake stewardship activities in accordance with international recommendations.[50] Indeed, the effect of the absence of authorities and resources in the face of the inherent complexity of global health governance has gained greater and greater traction in the global health arena. In particular, we are starting to see more of a role for formal and informal stakeholders (e.g., Wellcome Trust, Bill and Melinda Gates Foundation, World Bank, corporations) increasingly shaping and guiding global health activity through many channels – many of which are no longer transparent nor are the varied values and interests of these stakeholders always easy to fully comprehend.[51] As such, the super-wicked problem of AMR sits within a much broader complex challenge that

---

[47] See e.g. the World Health Organization's *Global Action Plan on Antimicrobial Resistance* (Geneva: WHO, 2015).

[48] P. Collignon, et al., 'Antimicrobial Resistance: The Major Contribution of Poor Governance and Corruption to this Growing Problem,' *PLoS One* 10(2015): e0116746; B. Rönnerstrand and V. Lapuente, 'Corruption and use of antibiotics in regions of Europe,' *Health Policy* 121(2017): 250–256.

[49] See World Health Organization, 'Interagency Coordination Group on Antimicrobial Resistance (IACG), https://www.who.int/antimicrobial-resistance/interagency-coordination-group/en/ (accessed October 10, 2018), and World Health Organization, *FAO, OIE, WHO – Tripartite Concept Note* (Geneva: WHO, 2010) http://www.who.int/foodsafety/areas_work/zoonose/concept-note/en/ (accessed October 10, 2018).

[50] B. Bennett and J. Iredell, "Global health governance and antimicrobial resistance" In *Ethics and Drug Resistance: Collective Responsibility for Global Public Health*. Springer, Cham.

[51] C. Clinton and D. Sridhar, *Governing Global Health* (Oxford: Oxford University Press, 2017); J. Youde. *Global Health Governance* (Cambridge: Polity Press, 2012); Nora Kenworthy, Ross

is making sense of, and impacting, global health governance, thus amplifying and multiplying the complexity of addressing AMR.

Criterion 4: Current Policies Discount the Future Irrationally

There is a notable disparity between the enormous significance that antibiotics have in today's health care systems and the lack of a comprehensive and realistically implementable global strategy to protect them as a resource for current and future generations.[52] Indeed, while the impact of AMR on health outcomes today and in the future is increasingly recognized, there remains a lack of coordination and sufficient funding to address the problem. When the health ministers of the G20 countries met for the first time in 2017, they declared "AMR has the potential to have a major negative impact on public health as well as on growth and global economic stability".[53] Other impact assessments have come to similar conclusions.[54] Since modern medicine relies so heavily on antibiotics as a prophylactic for standard surgical procedures, the further progression of AMR would be detrimental not only for infectious disease policy, it would also affect the outcome of surgical care or the survival chances of cancer patients. In short, AMR has become a wider health system issue.[55] It is therefore all the more surprising that current policies do not place greater emphasis on long-term strategies to preserve antibiotic effectiveness and best-case policy scenarios consist in the preservation of some level of antibiotic effectiveness in the short run, without a comprehensive replacement strategy for ineffective drugs.[56]

Due to the complexity of the drivers of AMR, its costs are extremely difficult to assess, even if they are only measured locally or in the short run.[57] A number of recent economic models have attempted to model the long-term costs, but due to the

MacKenzie, and Kelley Lee (eds.), *Case Studies on Corporations and Global Health Governance: Impacts, Influence and Accountability* (Rowman & Littlefield, 2016).

52 M. Millar M, 'Can antibiotic use be both just and sustainable... or only more or less so?' *Journal of Medical Ethics* 37(2011): 153–7; L. Leibovici, M. Paul and O. Ezra, 'Ethical dilemmas in antibiotic treatment,' *Journal of Antimicrobial Chemotherapy* 67(2012): 12–16.

53 Berlin Declaration of the G20 Health Ministers, Berlin 2017, p. 5 https://www.bundesgesundheitsministerium.de/fileadmin/Dateien/3_Downloads/G/G20-Gesundheitsministertreffen/G20_Health_Ministers_Declaration_engl.pdf (accessed on September 25, 2017).

54 O. Adeyi. et al., Drug-resistant infections: A threat to our economic future, Volume 2 (Washington, D.C: World Bank, 2017), available at http://documents.worldbank.org/curated/en/323311493396993758/final-report

55 R. Smith and J. Coast, 'The true cost of antimicrobial resistance,' *BMJ* 346(2013): f1493.

56 A.J. Alanis, 'Resistance to Antibiotics: Are We in the Post-Antibiotic Era?' *Arch Med Res* 36(2005): 687–705.

57 D.H. Howard, R.D. Scott, 'The Economic Burden of Drug Resistance,' *Clin Infect Dis* 41(2005): S283-S86; R. Smith and J. Coast, 'The true cost of antimicrobial resistance,' *BMJ* 346(2013): f1493.

complexity of AMR, they inevitably have to restrict their analysis to a select number of bacterial pathogens or consider a limited number of potential cost factors.[58] As a result, existing cost models likely underestimate the long-term effects of AMR. However, even these conservative cost models, which – by their own admission – systematically underestimate some of the costs associated with drug resistance, come to the conclusion that the cost of AMR (including resistance to antiviral drugs) may exceed $100 trillion in total GDP loss by 2050.[59] What this shows quite clearly is that current efforts to address AMR are simply not proportionate to the magnitude of the challenge at hand.

This also raises questions about the proportionality of our policy responses – in a moral and legal sense – in light of how it will be legitimate for us to act given the seriousness of the challenge faced. If the spread and magnitude of harm of AMR will be as predicted, what could be currently seen as a disproportionate response – for instance, what might be seen as overly paternalistic or coercive measures – may be seen to be justified as the problem worsens. Nevertheless, if the long game here is about keeping AMR at bay for as long as possible, should we actually have to wait until the problem gets much worse before we are justified in utilizing more paternalistic or coercive measures to achieve the same goal? The moral and legal calculus involved – and the extent to which the legitimacy of our responses should be determined in proportion to the risk of harm – could signal, for example, the development of new or more stringent stewardship obligations, the imposition of more risk on individuals (even without consent) and potential limitations on once established and uncontroversial entitlements and rights.[60] The nature of super-wicked problems are such that we must consider not only what norms and values should advance particular social, medical and public health goals, but also how such norms and values can set constraints or limits on these goals.

---

[58] J. Taylor, et al., *Estimating the economic costs of antimicrobial resistance: models and results* (Cambridge, UK: RAND Europe, 2014); KPMG, *The global economic impact of antimicrobial resistance* (London: KPMG: 2014).

[59] J. O'Neill et al., Tackling Drug-Resistant Infections Globally: Final Report and Recommendations. (London: Review on Antimicrobial Resistance, 2016), available at https://amr-review.org/sites/default/files/160518_Final%20paper_with%20cover.pdf (accessed September 29, 2017).

[60] Gro Harlem Brundtland, who served three terms as Prime Minister of Norway and as Director-General of the World Health Organization from 1998 to 2003, maintained that "AMR is just as much about human rights and justice as it is about health" [http://blogs.bmj.com/bmj/2017/12/06/gro-harlem-brundtland-new-who-guidelines-are-crucial-step-to-fighting-antimicrobial-resistance/]

How Conceptualizing AMR as a Super-Wicked Problem Can Inform Policy Making

The account of AMR as a super-wicked problem is not merely descriptive, but offers a framework for assessing the expected impact of policy making. Understanding AMR as a super-wicked problem underlines three important facts. First, it highlights the tendency of current policies to focus on preserving antibiotic effectiveness, while failing to reduce the future need for antibiotics. Second, it explains why traditional instruments, such as cost-benefit analysis (CBA), are unsuited to determining an appropriate policy response. Third, it helps bring to light how the complex interaction of ethical considerations will contribute to shaping which policy options will be viewed as acceptable.

Many of the existing policies that address AMR (and a considerable portion of the academic literature) emphasize the need for new antibiotics, as well as the cost-effective and prudent use of available resources.[61] The policy focus is thus on addressing problems on the supply side, and the creation of new resources, where a broad number of policy campaigns already exist.[62] However, if AMR is understood as a super-wicked problem, it becomes apparent that such approaches – while a necessary contribution – will ultimately and inevitably fall short of the goal of effectively controlling AMR in the long run. Consideration must take place of the relative value of focusing on upstream versus downstream determinants of drug-resistant infections, and the extent to which values other than efficiency or innovation (e.g., health equity) should guide both which drivers of resistance we focus on as well as which preventive and therapeutic responses we should pursue.

Framing AMR as a super-wicked problem should lead policy makers to place a much stronger emphasis on those policies, which – to paraphrase Levin et al. – generate a shift in path dependencies.[63] The concept of path dependencies explains current policies in light of their development of time, and as a result of earlier decision.[64] A given policy may therefore be more influenced by legacy decisions than by

---

[61] E. Mossialos, *et al*, *Policies and incentives for promoting innovation in antibiotic research* (Copenhagen: European Observatory on Health Systems and Policies, 2008); T. Groves, 'Back to basics with the three Rs,' *BMJ* 344(2012); R. Laxminarayan and G.M. Brown, *Economics of Antibiotic Resistance: A Theory of Optimal Use* (Washington D.C. Resources for the Future, 2001); C. Morel and E. Mossialos, 'Stoking the antibiotic pipeline,' *BMJ* 340(2010): c2115.

[62] L.D. Högberg, A. Heddini, and O. Cars, 'The global need for effective antibiotics: challenges and recent advances' *Trends Pharmacol Sci* 31(2010): 509–15.

[63] K. Levin, et al., 'Overcoming the tragedy of super wicked problems: constraining our future selves to ameliorate global climate change,' *Policy Sciences* 45(2012): 123–52.

[64] A more complete definition of path dependence is as follows: 'Path dependence is the idea that decisions we are faced with depend on past knowledge trajectory and decisions made, and are thus limited by the current competence base. In other words, history matters for current decision-making situations and has a strong influence on strategic planning… A well-known example is the QWERTY layout for typewriters. Despite the fact that different keyboard layouts in modern computer keyboards would allow faster typing, the QWERTY layout prevails.' *Financial Times Lexicon* http://lexicon.ft.com/Term?term=path-dependence (accessed September 30, 2017).

the current state of affairs and the latest available evidence. A shift in path dependencies is necessary once it has become apparent that the trajectory of earlier policy decisions is leading to an unsustainable outcome in the long run. In the case of climate change, for example, such path dependency is exemplified by the widespread and continued reliance on fossil fuels.[65] In the case of AMR, this path dependency is reflected by the reliance on antibiotics as not only a treatment against acute infection, but also as a tool for infection prevention in both clinical and veterinary settings. This dependency is replicated in most current policies that focus on pulling on the same levers, which aim at either increasing the availability of antibiotics or decreasing the use of antibiotics. What is crucially missing is sufficient emphasis on infection prevention and control measures that reduce the need for antibiotics in the first place.

Consequently, current policies do not offer a long-term fix to the problem of AMR and create, at best, a "faux paradigmatic change", in which the implementation of policy only makes small corrections to a previous policy failure temporarily.[66] The most obvious example for a faux paradigmatic shift is the reliance on future developments of new antibiotics, which are effective against resistant bacteria. While such a development will provide significant short-term improvements, past experience suggests that bacteria will ultimately develop resistance to new classes of antibiotics, as well. Consequently, as Spellberg has observed, "we will never truly defeat microbial resistance; we can only keep pace with it."[67] In the absence of a realistic option for true paradigmatic change (i.e., a technological method to avoid the further emergence and spread of AMR altogether), it appears advisable to abandon ambitions to outpace the adaptation of microbes to new antibiotics, and instead focus on the creation of incremental but transformative changes, which no longer follow the same policy trajectory and instead reduce the dependence on antibiotics. In particular, this new trajectory must have as a chief focus policy options that can be effectively implemented in LMICs.

One analogy that summarizes this situation, and which has been used repeatedly to describe the problem at hand, is that of a "leaky bucket".[68] If we think of antibiotic effectiveness as a resource contained in a bucket, the emergence of resistance is

---

[65] G. Unruh, 'Understanding Carbon Lock-In,' *Energy Policy* 28(2000): 817–30; P. Aghion, C. Hepburn, A. Teytelboym, and D. Zenghelis, *Path dependence, innovation and the economics of climate change* (London: Centre for Climate Change Economics and Policy Grantham Research Institute on Climate Change and the Environment, 2014) http://www.lse.ac.uk/GranthamInstitute/wp-content/uploads/2014/11/Aghion_et_al_policy_paper_Nov20141.pdf (accessed September 29, 2017).

[66] B. Cashore and M. Howlett, 'Punctuating Which Equilibrium? Understanding Thermostatic Policy Dynamics in Pacific Northwest Forestry,' *Am J Pol Sci* 51(2007): 532–51; K. Levin, et al. 'Overcoming the tragedy of super wicked problems: constraining our future selves to ameliorate global climate change,' *Policy Sciences* 45(2012): 123–52.

[67] H.W. Boucher, et al. 'Bad Bugs, No Drugs: No ESKAPE! An Update from the Infectious Diseases Society of America,' *Clin Infect Dis* 48(2009): 1–2.

[68] This analogy was originally proposed by Prof. Otto Cars, ReAct-Action on Antimicrobial Resistance, Uppsala University Sweden.

akin to holes in this bucket, slowly draining the effectiveness of available drugs. The development of a new drug would effectively add water to the leaking bucket. But, in the absence of a realistic option to develop antibiotics that avoid the subsequent emergence of resistance, this will only have a temporary effect and not address the underlying problem; namely, the holes in the bucket. Thus, not only are the antibiotics currently in clinical development not adequate to counter the increasing prevalence of AMR, it is unlike they ever could be.[69]

A second argument for framing AMR as a super-wicked problem is that this approach discourages a reliance on CBA in policy making. Super-wicked problems – by their nature – are not easily solvable with standard CBA tools because they describe scenarios in which the cost of inaction will be very high, yet occur at some point in the distant future. Consequently, CBA will usually recommend an insufficiently large commitment of resources to address super-wicked problems because costs incurred today are pitted against benefits at a later stage for which neither magnitude nor time frame are known.[70] As outlined earlier, existing cost-models for the assessment of the economic burden of AMR systematically underestimate the true cost of AMR because, as Smith and Coast argue, "[none] considered the bigger picture – a world in which there are no effective antibiotics for situations where they are currently used routinely".[71] And where it has been attempted to take these wider costs into consideration, the complexity of AMR has usually forced analysts to restrict their models to pathogens and geographical regions for which reliable data exists.[72] One response to this criticism of CBA in policy-making is to suggest that a bad estimate of cost is still better than no estimate at all. However, as Jamieson rightly points out, this response overlooks that whenever uncertainties about future developments are great, relying on the supposedly neutral judgment of a bad cost-estimate is a leap of faith – and it may prompt us to reach policy decisions that, in the long run, are far worse than the ones we might have considered had we not aimed for cost-efficiency based on unreliable or incomplete information.[73]

A final argument for framing AMR as a super-wicked problem is that this approach provides a greater prominence on the importance of the values and norms that should inform what would make particular policy options more or less

---

[69] World Health Organization, *Antibacterial Agents in Clinical Development: An Analysis of the Antibacterial Clinical Development Pipeline, including Tuberculosis* (Geneva: World Health Organization, 2017).

[70] R. Lazarus, 'Super wicked problems and climate change: restraining the present to liberate the future,' *Cornell Law Re*view 94(2009): 1153–234.

[71] R.D. Smith and J. Coast, 'The true cost of antimicrobial resistance'. BMJ 2013; 346: f1493. Also cf. J. Coast and R.D. Smith, 'Distributional Considerations in Economic Responses to Antimicrobial Resistance,' *Public Health Ethics* 8(2015): 225–237.

[72] See e.g. the RAND corporations cost model for O'Neill's AMR review: https://www.rand.org/pubs/research_reports/RR911.html (accessed September 29, 2017).

[73] D. Jamieson, 'Ethics, Public Policy and Global Warming,' in S.M. Gardiner, et al. (eds.) *Climate Ethics* (Oxford: Oxford University Press, 2010), pp. 77–86. Also cf. A. Williams, 'Cost-effectiveness analysis: is it ethical?' *Journal of Medical Ethics* 18(1992): 7–11.

acceptable.[74] Through diminishing an analysis of the cost of AMR in primarily economic terms, it helps bring to light the non-economic costs and values involved in shaping which policy options will be viewed as acceptable. By emphasizing the need for shifts in path dependencies, and the resultant changes in our approaches and responses, it also emphasizes the need to re-evaluate the values and norms which underpinned our previous policies and activities. To put it another way, through framing AMR as a super-wicked problem, we not only acknowledge that previous approaches are unlikely to be sustainable in the long run, but we are also forced to ask what sort of values and norms could justify new policy options that would not only be effective but also ethical. This is all the more relevant because understanding AMR as more than a scientific or technical issue is a relatively new perspective. For most of the existence of antibiotics, their use has been primarily viewed as a medical or microbiological issue, and was governed accordingly. This means that value judgments were commonly only implicit and often incoherent. We have seen that these technical or medical matters do not exhaust all of the relevant considerations, and much of the decision-making and policy-making around AMR concerned matters that were inherently and inescapably ethical. Acting as an antimicrobial steward, for instance, often involves making moral judgments, promoting particular values and prioritising different aims – which are normative, and not merely technical, activities. In viewing AMR as a societal challenge, we can see the failings of earlier approaches that had not considered the normative significance this shift implies.

Incrementally Creating Transformative Shifts in Path Dependency: Alternative Strategies

Creating transformative changes in path dependency will require adjustments on all types and levels of antibiotic use, and is unlikely to come in the shape of a single intervention. While there are no formulaic strategies to address wicked and super-wicked problems, different kinds of policy response will be suited to different time frames and address different aspects of the challenge that AMR presents. Nancy Roberts distinguishes between three possible approaches to super-wicked problems: authoritative, competitive and collaborative strategies.[75]

---

[74] For different ways in which framing the problem of AMR can have ethical and political implications, see, for instance, A.M. Viens and Jasper Littmann, 'Is Antimicrobial Resistance a Slowly Emerging Disaster?' *Public Health Ethics* 8(2015): 255–265.

[75] N. Roberts, 'Wicked Problems and Network Approaches to Resolution,' *Int Public Manag Rev* 1(2000): 1–19.

Authoritative Strategies

These strategies involve a small number of decision-makers who develop policy solutions, which are then implemented by others. Such approaches require that decision-makers have the ability to enforce the implementation of their chosen strategy. The advantage of such a policy is that decision-making complexity is reduced, and policies can be implemented and adjusted relatively quickly. On the other hand, such approaches to solving super-wicked problems are likely to alienate a large proportion of stakeholders and they depend on the existence of power structures where they can be enforced.[76] To this end, recent proposals for international legal frameworks and an intergovernmental panel have been put forward.[77] However, the question how adherence at the local level could be controlled and, where necessary, enforced – let alone sufficiently resourced – make such centralized and costly proposals very difficult to implement. Authoritative strategies may therefore be of greater use at the national or regional level. At the global level, however, the current lack of adequate resource, governance and accountability structures, which could help to effectively implement them, is likely to limit their usefulness in addressing the challenge of AMR.

Competitive Strategies

These strategies let different stakeholders or corporations compete for the creation of (market-based) solutions and often lead to creative approaches to problem solving.[78] However, the commitment of stakeholders will largely depend on the strength of incentives to focus on a given policy area. In the case of AMR, the absence of sufficient market incentives has led to minimal investments into R&D for new antibiotics, which lies well below a socially optimal level.[79] Recent initiatives such as

[76] L. Briggs, 'Tackling Wicked Problems – A Public Policy Perspective,' in *Contemporary Government Challenges* (Australian Public Service Commission, 2007).

[77] J. Anomaly, 'Combating Resistance: The Case for a Global Antibiotics Treaty,' *Public Health Ethics* 3(2010): 13–22; M. Woolhouse and J. Farrar, 'Policy: An intergovernmental panel on antimicrobial resistance,' *Nature* 509(2014): 555–557; Steven J. Hoffman, 'An international legal framework to address antimicrobial resistance,' *Bulletin of the World Health Organization* 93(2015): 66; S.J. Hoffman, J-A. Røttingen and J. Frenk, 'International Law Has a Role to Play in Addressing Antibiotic Resistance,' *Journal of Law, Medicine & Ethics* 43(2015): 65–67; A.D So, et al., 'An integrated systems approach is needed to ensure the sustainability of antibiotic effectiveness for both humans and animals,' *J Law Med Ethics*. 2015:43(Suppl 3):38–45; N. Gulati, et al., *Using International Instruments to Address Antimicrobial Resistance* (Ottawa: University of Ottawa Global Strategy Lab, 2016).

[78] N. Roberts, 'Wicked Problems and Network Approaches to Resolution,' *Int Public Manag Rev* 1(2000): 1–19.

[79] E. Mossialos, et al., *Policies and incentives for promoting innovation in antibiotic research* (Copenhagen: European Observatory on Health Systems and Policies, 2008).

the US Generating New Antibiotic Incentives Now (GAIN) Act or the European Innovative Medicines Initiative (IMI) are trying to address this, but even if successful, their overall budget does not permit any kind of paradigmatic shift to current antibiotic use policy.[80] Other strategies which have been offered, such as antibiotic de-linkage schemes,[81] health impact funds,[82] public-private partnerships,[83] innovation prizes[84] and other mechanisms[85] have mostly sought to replicate the old approach of developing new antibiotics in the hopes of outpacing resistance. While some AMR funding streams now include calls for projects in behavioral science, communication and education, their funding remains a miniscule fraction of what is currently being invested into drug development. From an ethical perspective, this creates additional problems. New drugs are likely to disproportionately benefit high-income countries (HICs), despite LMICs having the greatest burden of drug-resistant infections. Behavioural science research is also predominantly focused on HICs. We currently lack sufficient behaviour change research into what can be effectively achieved in regions with high levels of resistance and limited resources, e.g. some African countries, India, or countries in South East Asia. Competitive strategies are unlikely to change this as they are currently structured and incentivized.

Collaborative Strategies

These strategies involve a large number of stakeholders, especially in cases where responsibility and decision-making power are widely dispersed. While more difficult to establish than top-down authoritative approaches, collaborative strategies are widely considered to be the most suitable approach to dealing with wicked and

---

[80] J.P. Roberts, 'Incentives aim to boost antibiotic development,' *Nature Biotechnology* 30:8 (2012):735.

[81] C. Clift, et al. (eds.), *Towards a New Global Business Model for Antibiotics: Delinking Revenues from Sales* (London: Chatham House, 2015).

[82] K. Outterson, T. Pogge and A. Hollis, 'Combating Antibiotic Resistance Through the Health Impact Fund,' in I. Glenn Cohen (ed.), *The Globalization of Health Care: Legal and Ethical Issues* (Oxford: Oxford University Press 2013), pp. 318–338.

[83] For example, DRIVE-AB (Driving reinvestment in research and development and responsible antibiotic use), available from: http://drive-ab.eu; CARB-X (Combating antibiotic resistant bacteria biopharmaceutical accelerator), available from: http://www.carb-x.org

[84] For example, the Longitude Prize, available at: https://longitudeprize.org; Antimicrobial Resistance Diagnostic Challenge, available at: https://dpcpsi.nih.gov/AMRChallenge. Also see J. Love and T. Hubbard, 'The Big Idea: Prizes to Stimulate R&D for New Medicines,' *Chicago-Kent Law Review* 82(2007): 1519–1554.

[85] K. Outterson, J.H. Powers, G.W. Daniel, and M.B. McClellan, 'Repairing the Broken Market for Antibiotic Innovation,' *Health Affairs* 34(2015): 277–285; M.J. Renwick, D.M. Brogan and E. Mossialos, 'A Systematic Review and Critical Assessment of Incentive Strategies for Discovery and Development of Novel Antibiotics,' *The Journal of Antibiotics* 69(2016): 73–88; R.D. Smith, and J. Coast. 'The economics of resistance through and ethical lens,' In *Ethics and Drug Resistance: Collective Responsibility for Global Public Health*. Springer, Cham.

super-wicked problems, especially in the absence of a strong global planning authority to address the challenge.[86] Collaborative strategies can and are already being used at different levels, from UN initiatives to regional local campaigns that focus on raising awareness or improve prescribing.[87]

These three strategies are not mutually exclusive and different approaches can and should be combined, where viable and appropriate. Viewing AMR as a super-wicked problem suggests that sustainable change is most likely to result from collaborative strategies focusing on multiple drivers, yet the urgency with which a response to AMR must be found may necessitate, for example, the inclusion of competitive strategies to develop new drugs and authoritative strategies at the national level to enforce strict prescribing guidelines or prohibitions on using antibiotics in farm animals as growth promoters. However, the critical reader will also notice that, for the most part, present efforts to address AMR can already be categorized as authoritative, competitive or collaborative strategies respectively. This begs a question as to whether framing AMR as a super-wicked problem can be of any further help in developing novel and effective strategies to combat drug resistance. In the paper's penultimate section, we canvass a few potential ways in which the super-wicked problem frame can impact on current AMR policy going forward.

Shifting Path Dependencies – The Way Forward

Understanding AMR as a super-wicked problem itself does not, unfortunately, generate a set of novel, easily implementable policy solutions. Yet, as outlined before, the complexity of AMR, as well as the countless factors that contribute to it, make one-stop solutions highly unlikely in the first place.

While it does not offer any immediate solution to the problem, the understanding of AMR as a super-wicked problem may, however, achieve another goal – namely, to prompt a reconsideration of the relative importance of different responses to drug resistance. One of the most important insights of framing AMR as a super-wicked problem is that there is no technological fix we can engineer, nor any simple market-based solution that will avoid the impending scarcity of effective antibiotics in the future. Any responses that will help us keep AMR at bay in a significant way will involve a delicate balancing of benefits and burdens that will require difficult choices and restrictions to be imposed on individuals and populations. This insight is at odds with current research funding in the area of AMR, which is heavily skewed towards drug development.[88] Moreover, given the global scale of the problem, success in one

[86] L. Briggs, 'Tackling Wicked Problems - A Public Policy Perspectiv,' in *Contemporary Government Challenges* (series) (Australian Public Service Commission, 2007).

[87] For a selection of local initiatives see for example the ReAct Toolbox, https://www.reactgroup.org/toolbox/

[88] R. Kelly, et al., 'Public funding for research on antibacterial resistance in the JPIAMR countries, the European Commission, and related European Union agencies: a systematic observational analysis,' *The Lancet Infectious Diseases* 16(2016): 431–440.

part of the world will likely only be temporary, given the drivers brought and accelerated by globalization. Framing AMR as such a fundamentally unsolvable policy challenge may appear to be defeatist. However, the point is not to admit defeat, but to focus on those interventions that may be of greatest use in the long run – even if we can never overcome the vicious cycle of bacterial resistance and antibiotic obsolescence.[89] It may come as good news at this stage that many potential candidates for such a strategy already exist, but have simply not have been implemented properly.

The most obvious example in this context is infection control and prevention and water, sanitation and hygiene (WASH). While ultimately decisive for the control of nosocomial infections, hospital and healthcare hygiene and infection prevention have often appeared to be more of an afterthought in recent policy discussion. However, they remain of crucial importance for the prevention of infections, in both high- and low-income settings.[90] Similarly, many of the ongoing efforts for the creation of broader public awareness for the problem and causes of AMR have not yet achieved their desired goals.[91] Education and hygiene measures are no silver bullets – and have their own issues with compliance and recalcitrance – but if AMR is understood as a super-wicked problem, these policies should receive much greater recognition as a crucial part of an effective AMR strategy. Indeed, these are just some of the many different behaviour change interventions – aimed at both professionals and the public – that should comprise a multipronged and diversified response to AMR.[92] Of course, the success of such behavior change interventions will itself be dependent upon fixing even more fundamental problems plaguing global health, including poverty and extreme income inequality, since many

---

[89] A.E. Aiello, N.B. King and B. Foxman, 'Ethical Conflicts in Public Health Research and Practice Antimicrobial Resistance and the Ethics of Drug Development,' *American Journal of Public Health,* 96(2006): 1910–1914; B. Spellberg, J.G. Bartlett and D.N. Gilbert, 'The Future of Antibiotics and Resistance,' *New England Journal of Medicine* 368(2013): 299–302.

[90] S. Harbarth, et al., 'Antimicrobial resistance: one world, one fight!' *Antimicrobial Resistance and Infection Control* 4(2015): 49 – https://doi.org/10.1186/s13756-015-0091-2; Peter Collingon, et al., 'Anthropological and socioeconomic factors contributing to global antimicrobial resistance: a univariate and multivariable analysis,' *The Lancet Planetary Health* 2018; 2: e398–405. Also World Health Organization, *Guidelines on Sanitation and Health* (Geneva: WHO, 2018).

[91] Special Eurobarometer, *Antimicrobial Resistance Report, May – June 2013* (Brussels: EU Directorate-General Communication, 2013).

[92] See, for example, T. Edgar, S.D. Boyd and M.J. Palamé, 'Sustainability for behaviour change in the fight against antibiotic resistance: a social marketing framework,' *Journal of Antimicrobial Chemotherapy* 63(2009): 230–237; C.S. Lundborg and A.J. Tamhankar, 'Understanding and changing human behaviour—antibiotic mainstreaming as an approach to facilitate modification of provider and consumer behaviour,' *Uppsala Journal of Medical Sciences* 119(2014):125–133; Pubic Health England, *Behaviour Change and Antibiotic Prescribing in Healthcare Settings: Literature Review and Behavioural Analysis* (London: Public Health England, 2015); S. Tonkin-Crine, A.S Walker and C.C Butler, 'Contribution of behavioural science to antibiotic stewardship,' *BMJ* 2015; 350:h3413; K. Chaintarli et al., 'Impact of a United Kingdom-wide campaign to tackle antimicrobial resistance on self-reported knowledge and behaviour change,' *BMC Public Health* 16(2016):393.

technical and behavioral interventions are limited by adverse social, economic, and political contexts.[93] Tackling AMR will require those working in global health to directly address injustices, however one conceives of justice. Here, for our purposes, any conception of justice will do since the problem of injustices in global health are theoretically overdetermined.[94] In other words, practically speaking, tackling the levers that make AMR a super-wicked problem will have to include making real efforts to address global injustices for the various ways in which they contribute to the level of drug-resistant pathogens around the world.

Finally, understanding AMR as a super-wicked problem and thereby as a global challenge that defies simple solutions by any one party suggests that a much greater part of our efforts must be directed towards increasing standards of access and quality of prescribing in those regions where resources continue to be limited. We have not yet managed to ensure the provision of adequate access to antibiotics in many regions of the world, where the price of drugs is often prohibitive for patients and where over-the-counter sales have led to an unregulated and uncontrolled use of antibiotics.[95] We are, therefore, faced with a situation in which we have to reduce the excessive use of antibiotics in some regions of the world while ensuring greater access in others.[96] As Daulaire et al. maintain, 'meaningful access is dependent on good stewardship and vice versa.'[97] Nevertheless, this will require us to successfully confront and find answers to difficult distributive questions about when access should be increased or limited, and how to maintain sustainable fair access in a way that attempts to diminish the rate of AMR as long as possible. Stewardship to protect the effectiveness of antibiotics presupposes a functioning healthcare and legal system with sufficient oversight to regulate antibiotic usage adequately. New drugs, especially against Gram-negative bacteria, are badly needed and if resistance against drugs of last resort (e.g., carbapenems, colistin) further increases, we are officially out of options for treatment. In many of the countries that require greater access, it is difficult to guarantee even the most basic stewardship mechanisms. As a result, there is a need to explore different ways of approaching antibiotic governance in a global setting as part of responding to this super-wicked problem that genuinely

---

[93] S. Gill and I. Bakker, 'The global crisis and global health,' in S. Benatar and G. Brock (eds.), *Global Health and Global Health Ethics* (Cambridge: Cambridge University Press, 2011), pp. 221–238.

[94] See, for example, L. Reid "Antimicrobial resistance and social inequalities in health: considerations of justice" In *Ethics and Drug Resistance: Collective Responsibility for Global Public Health*. Springer, Cham, where the author provides an egalitarian argument toward this conclusion.

[95] R. Laximinarayan, et al. 'Antibiotic resistance – the need for global solutions,' *Lancet Infect Dis*, 13:12 (2013): 1057–98.

[96] G. Heyman, O. Cars, M.T. Bejarano, and S. Peterson, 'Access, Excess, and Ethics—Towards a Sustainable Distribution Model for Antibiotics,' *Upsala Journal of Medical Sciences* 119(2014): 134–141.

[97] Nils Daulaire, et al., 'Universal Access to Effective Antibiotics is Essential for Tackling Antibiotic Resistance,' *The Journal of Law, Medicine and Ethics* 43(2015): 17–21 at 18.

empowers local and regional stakeholders to shape the path dependencies that guide our response.

Conclusion

While AMR is a complex and arduous challenge, understanding it as a super-wicked problem does not mean it is intractable or that the multitude of drivers and stakeholders defy making substantial progress. The discussion of potential initiators of path dependency in this paper serves as an illustration of possible scenarios rather than as a comprehensive list of recommendations, but it highlights that recognizing AMR as a super-wicked problem would indeed have policy implications and should lead us to reconsider our values and priorities in responding to AMR.

This will also include a discussion of ethical norms and standards that should be met in addressing the problem of drug resistance. Given that AMR has only recently moved from being a purely clinical (or veterinary) problem into the realm of global challenges that require a broader societal response, there exists currently little research, and even less agreement on what the most important ethical issues in AMR are, and what we should do about them.[98] Ethicists should weigh in on such complex and wicked problems,[99] but they must also be aware of the fact that this is not an abstract problem, but already a health challenge on a global scale.

Understanding AMR as a super-wicked problem is not merely a matter of categorization. Instead, it should lead us to reconsider current policy approaches in light of their expected usefulness and likely success of implementation. New approaches to tacking AMR should seek to avoid replicating earlier patterns and problems of jumping between 'one-best-way' approaches or 'one-size-fits-all' interventions – both empirically and ethically. If AMR does indeed present a super-wicked problem, policy efforts should be primarily directed at shifting path dependencies. As such, the aim is not 'solving' AMR but to make progress towards better mitigation and management through these shifts. Current policies, for instance, which promote infection prevention and control, antimicrobial stewardship and the development of new drugs, are a crucial contribution to curbing AMR because they prolong antibiotic effectiveness and prevent infections in the first place. However, they are clearly insufficient as answers in the medium to long run, and should therefore only constitute a first step in initiating more fundamental changes to public health policy to reduce future dependence on antibiotics and more general social policy affecting the drivers of drug resistance.

---

[98] J. Littmann J and A.M. Viens, 'The Ethical Significance of Antimicrobial Resistance,' *Public Health Ethics* 8(2015): 209–224.

[99] D.S. Silva, M.J. Smith MJ, and C.D. Norman, 'Systems thinking and ethics in public health: a necessary and mutually beneficial partnership,' *Monash Bioethics Review* 2018 Jun 13. doi: https://doi.org/10.1007/s40592-018-0082-1. [Epub ahead of print].

Framing AMR as a super-wicked problem also emphasizes the importance of ongoing trends towards more integrated collaborations across sectors and research disciplines. It should help in creating greater awareness for the true scope of the problem we are faced with and the urgency with which we must address it.

Acknowledgements The authors would like to thank James Wilson and Anthony Kessel for feedback on an earlier draft of this paper.

13

Antimicrobial Footprints, Fairness, and Collective Harm

Anne Schwenkenbecher

Abstract This chapter explores the question of whether or not individual agents are under a moral obligation to reduce their 'antimicrobial footprint'. An agent's antimicrobial footprint measures the extent to which her actions are causally linked to the use of antibiotics. As such, it is not necessarily a measure of her contribution to antimicrobial resistance. Talking about people's antimicrobial footprint in a way we talk about our carbon footprint may be helpful for drawing attention to the global effects of individual behaviour and for highlighting that our choices can collectively make a real difference. But can we be morally obligated to make a contribution to resolving a collective action problem when our individual contributions by themselves make no discernible difference? I will focus on two lines of argument in favour of such obligations: whether a failure to reduce one's antimicrobial footprint is *unfair* and whether it constitutes wrongdoing because it is *harmful*. I conclude by suggesting that the argument from collective harm is ultimately more successful.

Keywords Political philosophy · Ethics · Public health · Antimicrobial resistance · Collective action problems

Introduction

Anti-microbial resistance and a decline in anti-microbial efficacy are urgent collective action problems. Who should act on this problem? According to the World Health Organisation's recommendations, concerted action on this issue requires efforts from a diverse array of actors: patients, drug prescribers and dispensers, hospitals, policy makers, and food producers (WHO 2001: 68–70, see also Littmann and Viens 2015).

A. Schwenkenbecher (✉)
Murdoch University, Perth, Western Australia
e-mail: A.Schwenkenbecher@murdoch.edu.au

In this chapter I explore the idea of an 'antimicrobial footprint' and discuss whether or not individual agents are under a moral obligation to reduce theirs. Importantly, I am not suggesting that reducing our antimicrobial footprints by way of individual behavioural change is the best or most efficient way of decelerating antimicrobial resistance, since that is an empirical question. However, given that the WHO identified individual agents such as patients and prescribers as agents of change, it seems that individuals' moral obligations deserve some discussion, which is why I will focus on those in this chapter. But before I do so, let me briefly point to another way in which individual agents are implicated in anti-microbial resistance: as consumers of products from animal industries. Notably, the aforementioned WHO report treats the implications of our aggregate meat consumption as an issue for regulation, but not one for individual behavioural change. In contrast, my argument includes individual consumer choices amongst the options individuals have for addressing antimicrobial resistance.

I will focus on two lines of argument for moral obligations to reduce one's antimicrobial footprint: whether a failure to reduce it is *unfair* and whether it constitutes wrongdoing because it is *harmful*. I conclude by suggesting that the argument from collective harm is ultimately more successful.

Antimicrobial Resistance as a Collective Moral Action Problem

Antimicrobial resistance is a collective action problem in that it is the result of many different agents' activities, it can only be solved by the concerted efforts of many different agents, and it seems rational for individual actors to free-ride because individual behavioural change (if taken in isolation) is neither responsible for the problem's occurrence nor could it ever remedy the problem.

Crucially, too, antimicrobial resistance is the *inevitable* result of using antimicrobials and thereby selecting microorganisms that are resistant to our drugs. Resistance will eventually emerge to any antimicrobial agent we use. This means that resistance as such is an effect that has to be factored into the 'good' that specific antimicrobials provide. To put it differently, it is only a matter of time for any antimicrobial drug to lose its efficacy. To undermine the public good of antimicrobial efficacy is to reduce overall efficacy and to produce resistance at a faster-than-necessary rate. Some have warned that we might be in danger of losing this public good altogether one day – a worst-case scenario, which we are currently capable of preventing. In order to do that, we need to slow down the process of emerging resistance through a more limited and more considerate use of such drugs.

But who is meant by 'we'? Unsurprisingly, many call for global regulation or even the socialization of the use of antibiotics in order to delay the erosion of this good (Smith and Coast 2002; Anomaly 2010). And no doubt, regulators, policymakers and industry leaders must be at the forefront of restricting the use of antimicrobials in a way that secures their continued efficacy.

But what about ordinary people – individual agents who consume antibiotics either directly (as patients) or indirectly (as consumers of animal products) or who prescribe them (as medical doctors)? The 'general community' was identified by the WHO as a target of intervention (WHO 2001). The assumption behind that seems to be that individual members of the general community *can* jointly reduce resistance. If that is the case, does it follow that we *ought to* do something about reducing resistance?

One of the starting points for answering this question is to establish what causal relationship obtains between our use of antibiotics and emerging resistance. According to WHO authors, "the relationship between use and resistance is not a simple correlation" when it comes to antimicrobials. "Paradoxically, underuse through lack of access, inadequate dosing, poor adherence and sub-standard antimicrobials may play as important a role as overuse" (WHO 2001: 15).

Further, it is not simply the case that those who are *causally* responsible for antimicrobial resistance are automatically *morally* responsible. That is, knowing how a problem came about, or which agent(s) caused it, does not necessarily tell us which agent(s) can be blamed for its occurrence or even who should fix it. *Retrospective moral responsibility* is often used synonymously with *moral blameworthiness*. The focus in this chapter will be on *prospective* – or *forward-looking* – *moral responsibility* in the sense of having a moral obligation to act or to bring about a certain outcome.

Clearly, any answer to the question of prospective moral obligations must be based on empirical data concerning which actions will really make a difference to antibiotic resistance. One of the great difficulties for making the case for moral obligations to change individuals' behaviour lies in the fact that no individual (human) agent's actions will make a measurable or perceptible difference to solving the problem. It is an issue on which only the aggregation and combination of countless individual actions and enduring behavioural change will have a real impact.

Both common-sense morality and traditional moral theory often struggle in dealing with collective moral action problems – cases where what is wrong or right cannot be determined by looking at individuals and their actions in isolation, but where instead these must be considered in conjunction or in aggregation. Increasingly, scholars are making an effort to rethink traditional ethical approaches with a view to better account for collective agents, actions and effects (May and Hoffman 1991; French and Wettstein 2006; French and Wettstein 2014; Hess et al. 2018). One of the early attempts to do so will be discussed further down: Derek Parfit proposed that we re-think our 'moral mathematics'. According to Parfit, we need to revise our notions of wrong and right, harm and benefit regarding aggregate effects, where individual actions only make a significant difference in conjunction with countless actions of others (Parfit 1984). It is easy to see that such collective moral action problems abound: Apart from anti-microbial resistance, climate change, and overfishing are cases that come to mind.

So who should act on these problems? The most obvious response would be to point to states and state agents and the need for new policies and regulation. And there is no doubt that such agents are in principle best suited for dealing with such complex large-scale problems. But there is a role for 'ordinary citizens' where governments fall short of doing what is required. Where climate change mitigation is concerned, for instance, the combined actions of individual agents can make a significant contribution to closing the so-called emissions gap, that is, the gap between the emission reductions countries have currently committed to and the reductions required for limiting global warming to a maximum of 2 °C (Dietz et al. 2009; Ostrom 2010; Wynes and Nicholas 2017).

Whether or not anti-microbial resistance is a problem that can be fixed or improved through the aggregate effect of individual behavioural change by patients and doctors, consumers and producers is ultimately an empirical question. But, in line with the *WHO Global Strategy for Containment of Antimicrobial Resistance,* I will proceed on the assumption that collectively individual actors can make a significant difference. Can this ground an obligation for patients, doctors, consumers and producers to make a joint effort towards reducing the use of antibiotics? In the following, I will re-assess some of the philosophical arguments defending ascriptions of individual obligations in combating collective action problems. I will introduce the idea of an 'antimicrobial footprint' and discuss whether not contributing to the public good of antimicrobial efficacy is unfair and whether or not it constitutes harmful behaviour. I will conclude by suggesting that not reducing your antimicrobial footprint (where it is possible for you to do so at an acceptable cost) is potentially wrong because it is harmful (even if your individual actions as such make no difference to antimicrobial resistance).

Antimicrobial Footprints

Let me start by introducing a new concept: that of an *antimicrobial footprint.* An individual agent's antimicrobial footprint would result from the extent to which her actions are causally linked to the use of antibiotics. The idea mirrors that of a carbon footprint, a measure which – however imperfect (Wright et al. 2011) – reflects the amount of greenhouse gases released into the atmosphere as a result of individuals' actions. Importantly, it links global effects to individual behaviour and highlights that our choices can collectively make a real difference. It may be a helpful tool, then, to start talking about our antimicrobial footprint in a way we talk about our carbon footprint.

With regard to antibiotics, a person's antimicrobial footprint would not necessarily be a measure of her contribution to resistance, but merely of her overall direct and indirect use. Direct use would involve using such drugs as a patient, prescriber or agricultural producer. Indirect use would involve the consumption of goods from animal industries that were produced by overusing antimicrobials. Our diet, then, plays a major role in accelerating resistance (Giubilini et al. 2017) (see also the chapter by Anomaly "Antibiotics and Animal Agriculture). It is important to note, though, that underuse of antibiotics also causally contributes to resistance, not just overuse.

To reiterate, the anti-microbial footprint is – just like one's carbon footprint – an imperfect measure. As mentioned above, the causal links between our use of antimicrobials and resistance are not always straightforward. But the concept as such draws attention to an important fact – that every single one of us is causally and morally implicated in the problem of antimicrobial resistance.

Note further that – just like with our carbon footprint – our antimicrobial footprint will differ depending on our needs and circumstances. If we live in a climate which forces us to heat or cool our dwellings during major parts of the year in order to be healthy and safe then our carbon footprint will necessarily be greater than that of a person living in a milder climate. Likewise, if we suffer from health conditions that require the use of antibiotics we will necessarily have a greater antimicrobial footprint. Reducing our carbon footprint as well as reducing our antimicrobial footprint must not involve unacceptable cost.

But just like in the case of greenhouse gas emissions, there are many instances where we can reduce our antimicrobial footprint at an acceptable cost. First, research shows that patients often ask for such drugs (and are prescribed such drugs) when it would not have been necessary (WHO 2001, see also chapter by Oakley). If doctors can avoid prescribing such drugs and patients stop insisting on them where they are not needed this can make a significant difference for the better.

Another way to reduce one's antimicrobial footprint at an acceptable cost (and with numerous co-benefits such as improved health) is to become vegetarian (or vegan) or at least to have a meat-reduced diet (or else to resort to game and fish caught in the wild). This is a factor that is missing from many public debates concerning antimicrobial resistance and also missing from the WHO report (2001) mentioned earlier.

Let us assume for the sake of argument that a reasonable way of promoting the idea of antimicrobial footprint reductions can be found – one which does not unduly jeopardize individuals' health and which promotes reductions that are truly effective. Do we have *moral obligations* to reduce our antimicrobial footprint? Why would anyone have such an obligation? The question is a serious one: by themselves, none of our individual antimicrobial footprint reductions would make a difference to local, or regional, let alone global antimicrobial efficacy. I call this the *impotence objection*, or the *no-effect-view*. The issue is a familiar one: can we be morally obligated to make a contribution to resolving a collective action problem when our individual contributions make no discernible difference? The view that we cannot be obligated to perform an action if it makes no discernible positive difference to a morally desirable outcome seems to be entailed by standard individualist act-consequentialism. The discussion of obligations to contribute to collective endeavours even where our individual actions make no perceptible difference is ongoing (Parfit 1984; Cullity 1995; Kagan 2011; Nefsky 2011; Schwenkenbecher 2014; Spiekermann 2014; Pinkert 2015).

I will not rehearse all positions here, nor even the main ones, but instead focus on two solutions that appear particularly interesting and suitable to the kind of problem we are faced with and which move outside the standard act-consequentialist framework: the argument from unfairness and the argument from collective harm (for a different argument based on solidarity, see chapter by Holm and Ploug "Solidarity and Antimicrobial Resistance"). Most importantly, these solutions avoid the problem of impotence or imperceptible effects by locating the wrongness of failing to contribute somewhere other than in the effects of one's individual actions.

The Argument from Unfairness

The first of these arguments is about fairness: Under certain conditions, it is unfair not to contribute to schemes that we benefit from, regardless of the immediate effect of our free-riding, that is, regardless of whether or not we undermine the scheme or make people worse off by defecting. According to Garrett Cullity's *Principle of Fairness* (Cullity 1995), if a person receives benefits from a scheme that satisfies the following conditions, it is unfair of her not to meet the requirements the scheme makes on those enjoying its benefits:

(i) The practice of participation in the scheme represents a net benefit for her;
(ii) Similarly, this practice does not make most others worse off either;
(iii) She is not raising a legitimate moral objection to the scheme. (p. 18f, paraphrased)

According to Cullity, the free-rider's unfairness lies in giving herself *objectionably preferential treatment* in such cases. The benefits she seeks to gain from free-riding "only exist because others who seek them take it upon themselves to contribute toward their production". In other words, her choice to free-ride is motivated by the benefits that others provide, while she grants herself the privilege of enjoying those benefits without providing them (1995: 22–23).

In a later paper, Cullity specifies that unfair actions are failures of *appropriate impartiality* (Cullity 2008). Judgments about fairness and unfairness concern actions for which one particular way of being impartial is morally required (2008: 3). "Unfairness requires not just that the impartiality you fail to display would have been appropriate, but that it is the appropriate way of doing what ought to be done, as it ought to be done." (2008: 5). Cullity gives the following general description of what is common to unfair actions:

"Not Φ-ing is unfair when:

(i) something ought, all things considered, to be done;
(ii) doing it as it ought to be done requires a form of impartiality;
(iii) Φ-ing is the appropriate form for that impartiality to take; and
(iv) the failure of appropriate impartiality can contribute to a non-instrumental explanation of the failure to do what ought to be done." (ibid.)

According to Cullity, then, what matters for assessing the wrongness of free-riding is not only whether there is an action that ought to be performed (or an outcome to be produced or a scheme to be implemented) but that there is a specific way in which this ought to be done, which requires people to apply some kind of impartial rule, rather than look to their own advantage. Doing "what ought to be done as it ought to be done" (ibid.) requires that individuals do not exempt themselves from contributing. That is, out of the two imperatives that bind agents in such cases – the imperative to produce the collective good and the imperative of distributive (or procedural) justice – the free-rider violates the latter even where she cannot be said to clearly violate the former (because she does not jeopardize the collective outcome with her defection alone).

How does this relate to our specific problem of antimicrobial footprint reductions? Let us assume that Cullity is correct in claiming that the above features characterise unfair actions. Is failing to reduce one's antimicrobial footprint unfair? In order for that to be true, it would have to be the case that reducing or limiting antimicrobial resistance is something that all-things-considered ought to be done. Such a claim implies that it can be done at an acceptable overall cost. I think we can safely assume that both are the case.

But what about doing it *as it ought to be done*? Is reducing our individual antimicrobial footprint the method by which we ought to combat anti-microbial resistance? Cullity rejects the idea that whenever a group ought to collectively act or produce a good, individual group members ought to be doing something to produce that good: "That would have odd implications for collective actions to which no one is contributing" (2008: 11). He thinks that it is not unfair if I do not unilaterally pursue a goal if there is no collectively agreed method for pursuing it (ibid.). Defecting (or exempting yourself from contributing to a collective good) is only unfair if there is such a method.

According to Cullity, a collectively agreed method for addressing a collective action problem is in place where the required course of action was decided in a fair procedure. He makes two qualifications though: first, that sometimes decisions produced by fair procedures can be bad and therefore need not to be respected. Second, that we may sometimes be obligated to respect the outcomes of procedures that though not perfectly fair are good enough. Unfortunately, Cullity does not specify what it means for a procedure to be good enough.

It is not possible here to have a detailed discussion on fair (or good enough) procedures for deciding on the production of collective goods. Regulation and legislation – where they result from legitimate democratic procedures – should arguably count as such. What is crucial for Cullity's procedural condition is the underlying rationale: that in order for a collective scheme to have legitimacy, in the sense that it gives individual agents binding reasons for playing their role therein, such a scheme must have been produced in the right way. If that is the case, then we as individual agents can be bound by rules (including laws) that are not of our own making and that we would in fact not have chosen ourselves. But these clarifications do not help with our current enquiry, since our focus is precisely on actions that are not called for by regulation and legislation, but on voluntary individual behavioural change that might be necessary while regulation and legislation fall short of reining in the problem.

This is the point where the fairness argument in favour of reducing our antimicrobial footprint crumbles, I believe. It is quite unclear what kind of method or procedure would count as fair where aggregate individual behavioural changes to reduce our use of antimicrobials are concerned. Would it be enough for such changes to have been recommended by an authoritative, politically neutral global body such as the WHO or other expert panels? According to WHO, its *Global Strategy for Containment of Antimicrobial Resistance* report is the result of expert consultation, workshops and consensus meetings. It is doubtful that this is the kind of procedure Cullity had in mind. Moreover, even though the panel has made recommendations for individual behaviour change, it has not in fact proposed an outright 'scheme' for individual participation with clearly defined roles and contributory actions. For both of these reasons, it does not constitute the kind of collective agreement that gives potentially binding reasons to individual agents. In sum, the argument put forward by Cullity cannot support the idea that individuals ought to take on a share in reducing antimicrobial resistance as a matter of fairness.

A different and more promising approach might be built on an argument that antibiotic overuse or misuse is a way of wronging others in that it harms those who suffer its consequences. This argument relies on a notion of 'collective' harm – a relatively new concept that is increasingly gaining traction.

The Collective Harm Argument

According to Elizabeth Cripps (2011), individual agents can be collectively responsible for harm brought about by their aggregate individual actions in some cases:

> a person becomes one of a group collectively responsible for harm once her contribution exceeds the amount such that, were everyone contributing only to that level, there would be no harm (p. 181)

In order for a person to be thus responsible for harm, certain conditions have to be met:

1. "individuals acted in ways which, in aggregate, caused harm, and which they were aware (or could reasonably be expected to have foreseen) would, in aggregate, cause harm (although each only intentionally performed his own act);
2. they were all aware (or could reasonably expected to have foreseen) that there were enough others similarly placed (and so similarly motivated to act) for the combined actions to bring about the harm; and
3. the harm was collectively avoidable: by acting otherwise (which they could reasonably have done), the individuals making up the putative group could between them have avoided the harm." (pp. 174f)

The crucial point to be noted is that in order to be *weakly collective responsible* (as Cripps puts it) for harm, individuals need to *know* (or be in a position to foresee) two things: (i) that if enough other people did what they do it will cause harm, and (ii) that there are enough other people doing what they do.

Whether or not a large enough number of people are in this position vis-à-vis antimicrobial resistance is an empirical question. However, I suspect that these epistemic conditions are not met when it comes to our antimicrobial footprint. The problem of antimicrobial resistance has much less presence in the media and public discourse than the problem of climate change and carbon footprint reductions, for instance.

Cripps' criteria are clearly modelled on Derek Parfit's (1984) conditions for collectively doing wrong or harming others. He, too, relies on an epistemic condition that is – currently – unlikely to be met where antimicrobial resistance is concerned:

> (C12) When (1) the outcome would be worse if people suffered more, and (2) each of the members of some group could act in a certain way, and (3) they would cause other people to suffer if *enough* of them act in this way, and (4) they would cause these people to suffer *most* if they *all* act in this way, and (5) each of them both **knows** these facts and **believes** that enough of them will act in this way, then (6) each of them would be acting wrongly if he acted in this way. (p. 81, my emphasis in bold)

According to both Cripps and Parfit, then, we only act wrongly if we know about the effects of our own antimicrobial overuse or misuse and we are aware that enough others are engaged in this practice. Consequently, public awareness campaigns would make it the case that Cripps' and Parfit's conditions are met. Public knowledge – which obtains where most people know some proposition to be true and most people know that most people know – would turn harmless actions into harm. But still, on their accounts there is – currently – no harm or wrongdoing committed by many if not most of those who contribute to antimicrobial resistance. Also, for Cripps, weakly collective responsibility does not imply that any individual has direct duties to avert the (aggregate) harm. Instead such duties fall to the group, first and foremost. That is, even if we were collectively responsible for antimicrobial resistance we would not be required to individually reduce our antimicrobial footprint on her account.

Let me now turn to Judith Lichtenberg, who combines the unfairness argument and the argument from aggregate harm (2010): If we knowingly contribute to harms that "depend on the joint effects of many people's actions" (p. 568) we accept that if a sufficient number of other persons act in the same way, these harms will occur. She thinks that to do so is wrong because it means to act *unfairly*: "In the case of aggregate harms, doing the right thing involves an appeal to the unfairness of acting inconsistently with how one thinks others ought to act." (2010: 569). As I understand Lichtenberg, contributing to aggregate harms is not *intrinsically* wrong, but is wrong because it cannot be justified in rule-consequentialist terms or by way of universalizing. Similar to Cullity, she argues that the wrongness lies in exempting oneself from a rule that one should accept as morally optimal.

Note that Lichtenberg's account is more demanding than Cripps' and Parfit's because it does not have as strong a knowledge condition. For the wrongness of contributing it does not matter whether or not an individual agent knows that enough others will perform the same action and harm will be thus caused in aggregation. It suffices for the individual to know that collectively we should adopt a rule prohibiting such actions. This is a more demanding account because it seems to require us (*pro tanto*, at least) to individually refrain from doing what is collectively suboptimal. As I understand it, Lichtenberg's rule, if applied to antimicrobial footprint reductions, would imply that avoidable antimicrobial overuse and misuse are instances of harming, from which we (*pro tanto*) ought to abstain.

In response, one might argue that to demand – as Lichtenberg appears to do – that we individually do our part in a pattern that is collectively optimal is too strong a requirement. After all, sometimes it may be right to do what is collectively suboptimal if no one else does what is collectively optimal and our individual 'sacrifice' would be pointless. However, note that if Lichtenberg's proposal is safe from this objection as long as it is understood as generating pro tanto obligations to avoid contributing to collective harm, that is, obligations that can be overridden by other, more important obligations. If the collective defection rate is too high, my *pro tanto* obligations may simply fail to become all-out obligations. That is, if not enough others contribute, I may not have an all-things-considered obligation to avoid collective harm.

Conclusion

In this chapter I discussed arguments in favour of a moral obligation to reduce one's individual antimicrobial footprint. Despite the intuitive appeal of this idea, there exists no simple, straightforward defence of an obligation to change our individual behaviour. High levels of collective awareness and a genuine collective willingness to address the problem of anti-microbial resistance appear to be important preconditions for motivating (all-out) obligations for individuals to reduce their antimicrobial footprint. It is one of the most frustrating aspects of collective action problems that it is precisely the publicly known lack of commitment to resolving them which seems to sustain and justify a (further) lack of commitment for all those who could potentially resolve it.

Acknowledgements The author gratefully acknowledges the financial support received from the Oxford Martin School for this project as a Visiting Fellow to the program "Collective Responsibility for Infectious Diseases" (April – July 2017) as well as the extremely valuable feedback from colleagues in the Oxford Martin School and the Uehiro Centre for Practical Ethics.

References

Anomaly, J. 2010. Combating resistance: The case for a global antibiotics treaty. *Public Health Ethics* 3 (1): 13–22.

Cripps, E. 2011. Climate change, collective harm and legitimate coercion. *Critical Review of International Social and Political Philosophy* 14 (2): 171–193.

Cullity, G. 1995. Moral free riding. *Philosophy and Public Affairs* 24 (1): 3–34.

———. 2008. Public goods and fairness. *Australasian Journal of Philosophy* 86 (1): 1–21.

Dietz, T., G.T. Gardner, J. Gilligan, P.C. Stern, and M.P. Vandenbergh. 2009. Household actions can provide a behavioral wedge to rapidly reduce US carbon emissions. *Proceedings of the National Academy of Sciences* 106 (44): 18452–18456.

French, P.A., and H.K. Wettstein, eds. (2006). Special Issue: Shared intentions and collective responsibility, Midwest Studies in Philosophy 30.

———, eds. (2014). Special issue: Forward-looking collective responsibility, Midwest Studies in Philosophy 38.

Giubilini, A., P. Birkl, T. Douglas, J. Savulescu, and H. Maslen. 2017. Taxing meat: Taking responsibility for one's contribution to antibiotic resistance. *Journal of Agricultural and Environmental Ethics* 30 (2): 179–198.

Hess, K.E., V.E. Igneski, and T.L.E. Isaacs. 2018. *Collectivity: Ontology, ethics, and social justice*. London: Rowman & Littlefield International.

Kagan, S. 2011. Do I make a difference? *Philosophy & Public Affairs* 39 (2): 105–141.

Lichtenberg, J. 2010. Oughts and cans. *Philosophical Topics* 38 (1): 123–142.

Littmann, J., and A.M. Viens. 2015. The ethical significance of antimicrobial resistance. *Public Health Ethics* 8 (3): 209–224.

May, L., and S. Hoffman. 1991. *Collective responsibility: Five decades of debate in theoretical and applied ethics*. Rowman & Littlefield: Savage.

Nefsky, J. 2011. Consequentialism and the problem of collective harm: A reply to Kagan. *Philosophy & Public Affairs* 39 (4): 364–395.

Ostrom, E. 2010. Polycentric systems for coping with collective action and global environmental change. *Global Environmental Change* 20 (4): 550–557.

Parfit, D. 1984. *Five mistakes in moral mathematics. Reasons and persons*. Vol. 1, 55–83. Oxford: Clarendon Press.

Pinkert, F. 2015. What if I cannot make a difference (and know it). *Ethics* 125 (4): 971–998.

Schwenkenbecher, A. 2014. Is there an obligation to reduce one's individual carbon footprint? *Critical Review of International Social and Political Philosophy* 17 (2): 168–188.

Smith, R.D., and J. Coast. 2002. Antimicrobial resistance: a global response. *Bulletin of the World Health Organization* 80: 126–133.

Spiekermann, K. 2014. Small impacts and imperceptible effects: Causing harm with others. *Midwest Studies In Philosophy* 38 (1): 75–90.

World Health Organisation. (2001). WHO global strategy for containment of antimicrobial resistance.

Wright, L.A., S. Kemp, and I. Williams. 2011. 'Carbon footprinting': Towards a universally accepted definition. *Carbon Management* 2 (1): 61–72.

Wynes, S., and K.A. Nicholas. 2017. The climate mitigation gap: Education and government recommendations miss the most effective individual actions. *Environmental Research Letters* 12 (7): 074024.